# NEUROPATHIC PAIN

Edited by **Cyprian Chukwunonye Udeagha**

**Neuropathic Pain**
Edited by Cyprian Chukwunonye Udeagha

**Published by InTech**
Janeza Trdine 9, 51000 Rijeka, Croatia



**Publishing Process Manager** Maja Bozicevic

**Technical Editor** Teodora Smiljanic

**Cover Designer** InTech Design Team

Additional hard copies can be obtained from orders@intechopen.com

Neuropathic Pain, Edited by Cyprian Chukwunonye Udeagha
p. cm.
ISBN 978-953-51-0452-0

For EU product safety concerns:
IN TECH d.o.o., Prolaz Marije Krucifikse Kozulić 3, 51000 Rijeka, Croatia,
info@intechopen.com or visit our website at intechopen.com.

# Meet the editor

Dr. Cyprian Chukwunonye Udeagha is presently Safe-employed General Practitioner and Pain Management Specialist. He had his primary education at Christ the King Primary School and post-primary education at Comprehensive Secondary School both in Aba Abia State. He attended the College of Medical Sciences, University of Maiduguri in Nigeria. With Bachelor of Medicine, Bachelor of Surgery (MBBS) in 1985 from the University of Maiduguri, he has the following postgraduate qualifications including Masters in Pain Management (MSc Pain) in 2007 from the University of Leicester, Professional Diploma in Tropical Child Health (Paediatrics) in 2003 from the School of Tropical Medicine, University of Liverpool and a Post-Graduate Certificate in Public Health, Merlin, London. Dr. Cyprian Chukwunonye Udeagha plays tennis and travel a lot.

# Contents

# Preface

Neuropathic pain is known to be pain with nerve involvement. The intensity of which depends on the severity, pain threshold and the ability of suffers to cope. Neuropathic pain may need mono-therapy or combination of therapies to be resolved. Neuropathic pain may not resolve completely, therefore patient's compliance and understanding is essential in its management. Awareness and patient's education on targets may be of help during therapies for neuropathic pain.

Unsatisfactory results from managements of neuropathic pain and unusual characteristics of neuropathic pain demand different methods for management of neuropathic pain. Such qualities have necessitated search for efficient and cost effective management of neuropathic pain. These involve research in pharmacological and non-pharmacological methods. All chapters treated introduction, characteristics, diagnosis and randomized interventions to certain management of neuropathic pain. We acknowledge all those involve in the making of this book

**Dr. Cyprian Chukwunonye Udeagha**
Zankli Medical Centre, Abuja,
Nigeria

# 1

# Overview of Neuropathic Pain Diagnosis and Assessment – An Approach Based on Mechanisms

Ioana Mindruta, Ana-Maria Cobzaru and Ovidiu Alexandru Bajenaru
*University Emergency Hospital of Bucharest*
*Romania*

## 1. Introduction

Neuropathic pain syndromes are, in the majority of cases, chronic conditions related to injuries or diseases occurring at different levels in the nervous systems which are involved in signaling pain. (Treede et al., 2008)

Regarded as heterogeneous states, usually these conditions could not be explained by a single cause or a single specific lesion. Many of these syndromes are expressed by the same clinical symptoms in different etiologies (e.g touch-evocated pain exists in both post herpetic neuralgia and painful diabetic neuropathy) and could be based on the same mechanism. However in the same disease, one mechanism may produce painful symptoms that take different aspects. (Gilron et al., 2006)

As neuroplastic changes occur in different structures of the nervous system, the distribution of pain will no longer respect nerves, roots, segments, proximal or distal territories. (Finnerup et al., 2006)

Recent advances in the field of pain mechanisms produced increasing evidences that old classifications based on underlying disease or anatomic grounds (see table 1) provide insufficient, arguments for the therapeutic approach. (Dworkin et al., 2003; Baron, 2006; Baron et al.. 2010).

Therefore, we discuss in this chapter whether a different strategy, in which pain is analyzed on the basis of underlying mechanism, could provide an alternative approach for diagnosis of patients suffering from neuropathic pain conditions with the aim of obtaining a better treatment outcome.

Quantitative sensory testing applied on 1236 patients suffering from different neuropatic pain conditions revealed that despite the heterogeneity in etiology and anatomical distribution, neuropathic pain is characterized by certain clinical features (Maier et al., 2010):

- widespread pain otherwise unexplainable;
- burning continuous spontaneous pain;
- sudden, unprovoked attacks of pain;
- evoked pain (stimulus dependent);
- pain located in a neuroanatomical area with partial or complete sensory deficit;
- aftersensations;

- abnormal summation of pain;
- sympathetic involvement.

<table>
<tr><td rowspan="2">Peripheral neuropathic pain syndromes</td><td>Focal and multifocal neuropathies</td><td>Phantom pain, nerve partial or complete transection pain, neuroma, entrapment syndromes, postherpetic neuralgia, diabetic mononeuropathy, ischemic neuropathy, plexopathies (radiation, diabetic, infiltrative, idiopathic, hereditary), trigeminal or glossopharyngeal neuralgia, vascular compression</td></tr>
<tr><td>Generalized neuropathies (polyneuropathies)</td><td>Metabolic or nutritional<br>Diabetes, amyloidosis, hypothyroidism, beri beri, pellagra<br>Drug-related<br>Antiretrovirals, cisplatin, oxaliplatin, thalidomide, vincristine, methylthiouracil, disulfiram, ethambutol, isoniazid, nitrofurantoin, chloramfenicol, metronidazol, taxoids, gold<br>Toxin-related<br>Thallium, arsenic, acrylamide, ethylene oxide, dinitrophenol, penthachlorofenol<br>Hereditary<br>Amyloid neuropathy, Fabry's disease, hereditary sensory and autonomic neuropathy type 1<br>Paraneoplastic syndromes<br>Paraneoplastic peripheral neuropathy<br>Infective or post-infective, immune<br>Acute inflammatory polyradiculoneuropathy, HIV, borreliosis<br>Other<br>Idiopathic small-fibers neuropathy, erythromelalgia</td></tr>
<tr><td>Central neuropathic pain syndromes</td><td colspan="2">Vascular lesion in the brain (frequently in the brainstem and thalamus) and spinal cord<br>Inflammatory diseases: multiple sclerosis and other<br>Traumatic spinal cord and brain injury<br>Tumors<br>Abscesses<br>Syringomyelia and syringobulbia<br>Parkinson disease</td></tr>
<tr><td>Mixed pain syndromes</td><td colspan="2">Chronic low back pain with radiculopathy<br>Complex regional pain syndromes<br>Cancer pain with malignant plexus invasion</td></tr>
</table>

Table 1. Neuropathic pain classification based on anatomy and underlying disease (modified from Baron R. et al., 2010)

These symptoms may occur in various combinations, but do not necessarily have to be present all together. The association of symptoms and signs is compatible with the process of general sensitization of the second and third order neurons in the central nervous system. These relay structures have lost part of their normal input that has been substituted by an altered afferent influx. Commonly, the process of sensitization is considered to be an essential phenomenon that explains persistent neuropathic pains. (Baron, 2006; Baron et al., 2010).

New insights regarding the pathophysiological mechanisms behind spontaneous and evoked phenomena were substantiated by experimental studies in animal models and clinical trials. The most relevant for clinical practice are:

- lesion in a peripheral nerve induce **ectopic activity in the primary nociceptive afferent fibers** both in injured and intact terminals. Alteration of ion-channels and up-regulation of a certain receptor proteins in the peripheral nociceptive endings are responsible for spontaneous pain as well as for allodynia and hyperalgezia that might evolve in the area innervated by the nerves with ectopic activity. (Wu et al. 2002; Amir et al. 2005).
- the local inflammatory reaction following a certain injury and exposure of the nerve terminals to the so called "inflammatory soup" may also lead to molecular changes in nociceptive neurons that will became abnormally sensitive, developing spontaneous pathological activity that contribute to **peripheral sensitisation**. This process is correlated with spontaneous and evoked pain and could occur even without any underlying nerve damage. (Finnerup et al. 2006)
- hyperactivity in the nociceptors lead to secondary changes in neurons processing somatosensory information in the dorsal horn, spinal cord and brain. Hence the input from the mechanoreceptive A beta, A delta fibers might activate second order neurons and hence, non innocuous stimulation could became painful. This process is called **central sensitization** and could be responsible for the central pain syndromes as well.(Baron , 2006; Finnerup et al. 2006).
- **loss of inhibitory interneurons** in the dorsal horn and brain stem in the context of neuroplastic changes may lead to alteration in segmental and descending modulation. Synaptic activity changes in the dorsal horn of the spinal cord thereby results in hyperexcitability of the second order neurons due to alteration of inhibitory control. This mechanism may mediate mechanical and thermal hyperalgezia. (Moore et al. 2002; Scholz et al. 2005).
- hyperactivity at the level of sensitized nociceptors that favor pain persistence and allodynia are correlated with **increasing activity in the sympathetic nervous system.** Spontaneous pain and dynamic mechanical hyperalgesia might get enhanced by the secondary changes in the sympathetic activity. This process could be interfered by sympathetic blocks. (Zhuo et al. 2011)
- **activation of the glial cells in the dorsal horn,** in the context of neuropathic pain conditions, is demonstrated to be responsible for neuronal hyperexcitability. Thus microglial cells are activated during the initial stages as well as the astrocites are more involved in the process of pain maintenance. (Boucsein et al.2000; Ji et al 2007; Gosselin et al. 2010)
- **cortical maps reorganization and the role of mirror neurons** in the brain have been proposed in the generation of phantom limb pain. (Subedi et al. 2011)

## 2. Diagnosis

The neuropathic pain represents a devastating condition that can be diagnosed by taking a relevant history of pain and by adequately performed neurological examination. Complementary studies, including blood and serologic tests, electrophysiological studies, imaging procedures will contribute with information about the etiology of the underlying disease and also to predict the outcome. (Gilron et al.2006; Haanpaa et al 2011).

Although the neuropathic pain is seen as a chronic condition, there are situations, poorly recognized, of acute neuropathic pain. Despite the fact that acute pain is perceived as having a nociceptive nature, in a small percent of cases, the pain is mixed, including a neuropathic component as well (e.g. acute disc herniation, postsurgery pain). Even if the incidence of acute neuropathic pain in acute pain services is low (1-3%), its importance resides in the high risk to progress to a persistent and debilitating status. Time interval which defines acute neuropathic pain is 6-12 weeks. (Hayes et al., 2002; Gray, 2008)

The nociceptive, neuropathic and mixed pains are the three main types of pain. The first one is induced by injured tissue, the second one is caused by a disorder in the somatosensory system and the third one refers to coexistence of the first two. To diagnose neuropathic pain and to differentiate it from the nociceptive type, or to identify the nociceptive component of the mixed condition, it is mandatory to analyze in detail the type of somatosensory abnormalities in a given case. By contrast with other neurological symptoms and signs (e.g motor deficit) pain as a subjective sensory symptom is difficult to measure because it is not something visible and does not involve only physical aspects, but also psychological and emotional components. (Baron et al 2010)

### 2.1 Interview and questionnaires

The first step in pain diagnostic and evaluation is a very detailed history with:

- description of qualities of pain;
- duration of pain;
- time course pattern;
- rating intensity of pain;
- the context and type of onset;
- presence of relieving factors;
- existence of provocative or enhancer factors;
- topographic distribution of pain;
- coexistence of other positive symptoms such as paresthesia;
- impact on daily activities and sleep.

Standardized screening tools have been developed to distinguish neuropathic pain on the basis of patient reported verbal descriptors of pain during the interview and a limited bedside examination. The purpose of these questionnaires is to identify the patients with neuropathic pain and also to distinguish between different pathophysiological groups. Some of these screening tools include items that refer to rating scales, time course pattern and topographical distribution. This particular aspect may help the examiner to find out if pain distribution respects a nerve or root territory. Moreover, the rating scales are also useful to monitor the efficacy of different therapeutic interventions (Cruccu et al., 2004; Haanpaa et al, 2011).

LANSS (Leedes Assessment of Neuropathic Symptoms and Signs Scale) is the first tool developed more for the diagnosis of neuropathic pain than for its rating(9) and consists of five items for description of symptoms and two items for clinical examination. Although it was not designed for measurement, LANNS proved its sensitivity to treatment. This tool has been subsequently tested and validated in several settings with sensitivity and specificity ranging from 82% to 91% and 80% to 94% respectively, comparing with clinical diagnosis. There is also a version of a self-report questionnaire, S-LANNS (Bennett, 2001).

NPQ (Neuropathic Pain Questionnaire) consists of twelve items of which ten refer to sensations and sensory responses and two are related to affect. NPQ has showed a sensitivity of 66% and a specificity of 74% versus clinical diagnosis. There is, also, a short variant that has only 3 items for similar discriminative properties (tingling, numbness and increasing pain in response to touch) (Krause et al., 2003).

DN4 (Douleur Neuropathique en 4 questions) is a questionnaire initially developed and validated in French and consists of seven items related to symptoms, which can be used as a self-report, and three items related to clinical examination. This tool is easy to use and a total score of 4 out of 10 or more suggests neuropathic pain. The DN4 proved 83% sensitivity and 90% specificity when compared with clinical diagnosis (Bouhassira et al., 2005).

ID-Pain does not require a clinical examination and was designed rather to screen for the presence of a neuropathic component. It consists of five sensory descriptor items with one item asking whether the pain is located in the joints (to identify nociceptive pain). In the validation study, 22% of patients in the nociceptive group, 39% in the mixed group and 58% in the neuropathic pain group scored above 3 points, the recommended cut-off score. (Portenoy, 2006).

PainDetect was developed and validated in a multicenter study conducted in Germany and includes seven weighted sensory descriptor items (from never to very strongly), two items relating to spatial (radiating and topography) and temporal characteristics of individual pain pattern and does not require clinical examination. This questionnaire showed a sensitivity of 85% and a specificity of 80% (Freynhagen et al., 2006).

Neuropathic Pain Scale (NPS) was designed and only preliminary validated in 1997 for evaluation of neuropathic pain symptoms (18). Although NPS has proved some sensitivity to treatment, it is no clear whether is adapted to detect differential effects of treatment on neuropathic symptoms. It consists in twelve items, self-reported, about the intensity and quality of pain (Galer et al., 1997).

Neuropathic Pain Symptoms Inventory (NPSI) includes ten descriptors and two items about temporal pattern of pain, that allow to differentiate and quantify five distinct features, clinically relevant, and sensitive to treatment. The questionnaire could be used to identify subgroups of patients with neuropathic pain characterized by specific clusters of symptoms and to verify if they respond in a different way to various pharmacological agents. The most important feature of this tool is the sensitivity to treatment variables (Bouhassira et al., 2004).

Standardized Evaluation of Pain (StEP) combines sixteen questions in the interview and twenty-three standardized clinical tests to evaluate symptoms and signs related to pain and to differentiate between various pain phenotypes reflecting distinct mechanisms. Scholz and colleagues evaluated the diagnostic utility of StEP in patients with low back

| Symptoms | Definition | Bedside exam | Expected pathological response | Mechanism(s) |
|---|---|---|---|---|
| Spontaneous sensations or pain | | | | |
| Paresthesia | Non-painful abnormal sensation | Grade intensity(0-10) | - | Spontaneous activity in low threshold A-β afferent |
| Dysesthesia | Unpleasant but non-painful abnormal sensation | Grade intensity(0-10) | - | Spontaneous activity in C/A-δ afferents |
| Paroxysmal pain | Attacks for seconds of shooting, stabbing or electric shock-like | Number, Grade(0-10) | - | Spontaneous activity in C-nociceptors |
| Superficial burning pain | Permanent pain located in the skin often of burning quality | Grade(0-10) | - | Spontaneous activity in C-nociceptors? |
| Deep pain | Permanent pain located in the muscles, bones, or internal organs | Grade(0-10) | - | Spontaneous activity in joint/muscle nociceptors? |
| Sympathetic maintained pain | Sustained burning pain associated with vasomotor, sudomotor and trophic changes on skin | Grade(0-10) | - | Peripheral sensitization: sympathetic-afferent coupling |
| Evoked pain | | | | |
| Dynamic allodynia provoked by mechanical stimulation | Pain provoked by normally non-painful light-pressure moving stimuli on skin | Stroking skin with painter's brush, cotton swab or gauze<br><br>Grade(0-10) | Sharp burning superficial pain in the primary affected zone, spreading into unaffected skin areas(secondary zone) | Central sensitization: A-β fibers input |

| | | | | |
|---|---|---|---|---|
| Mechanical static hyperalgesia | Pain provoked by normally non-painful gentle static pressure stimuli on skin | Apply gentle mechanical pressure to skin<br><br>Grade(0-10) | Dull pain presented in the area of affected primary afferent nerve endings (primary zone) | Peripheral sensitization |
| Mechanical punctuate or pin-prick hyperalgesia | Pain provoked by normally stinging but non-painful stimuli | Prick skin with a safety pin, sharp stick or stiff von Frey hair<br><br>Grade(0-10) | Sharp superficial pain presented in the primary affected zone, but spreads beyond into unaffected skin areas (secondary zone) | Central sensitization: A-δ fibers input |
| Temporal summation | Increasing pain sensation (wind-up-like pain) from repetitive application of identical single noxious stimuli | Prick skin with safety pin at intervals of 3 s for 30 s<br><br>Grade(0-10) | Sharp superficial pain of increasing intensity | Central sensitization: A-δ fibers input |
| Aftersensation | Pain occurred during the stimulation and persists more then seconds after stimulus cessation | Grade(0-10)<br>Duration | Persistent evoked pain | Central sensitization |
| Cold hyperalgesia | Pain provoked by non-painful cold stimuli | Contact skin with objects of 20° C for 10 s<br><br>Grade(0-10) | Painful burning temperature sensation presented in the area of affected primary afferent nerve endings (primary zone) | Peripheral sensitization with reduced activation threshold to cold |
| Heat hyperalgesia | Pain provoked by non-painful heat stimuli | Contact skin with objects of 40° C for 10 s<br><br>Grade(0-10) | Painful burning temperature sensation presented in the area of affected primary afferent nerve endings (primary zone) | Peripheral sensitization with reduced activation threshold to heat |

Table 2. Definitions and assessment of sensory symptoms in patients with neuropathic pain (modified from Baron et al., 2010)

pain. The StEP identified the radicular pain with 92 % sensitivity and a specificity of 97% (Scholz et al., 2009).

One of the most important aspects in the patient's interview is whether the pain is spontaneous or stimulus depended.

The spontaneous pain can be continuous or paroxysmal. In case of continuous neuropathic pain, the most common verbal descriptor used by patients to describe its quality is "burning". There are also other words the patients have used to describe their pain as a cold (frozen) sensation, stinging, electric shock, painful pins and needles, dull, squeezing, shooting, stabbing, cramping, throbbing, sharp, or pulling. Episodic or paroxysmal type of pain is usually lasting for seconds and is described as a shooting, electric, shock-like or stabbing sensation.

A thorough interview can reveal different types of evoked pain (hyperalgesia, allodynia). Thus painful symptoms could be provoked by light touch, mild pressure, heat or cold and also might be associated with the presence of an aftersensation phenomena. Hyperalgesia (an increased response to noxious stimuli by lowering the pain threshold) and allodynia (pain due to non-noxious stimulus) are typical elements of neuropathic pain.

The stimulus-evoked pain is further classified according to the stimulus type (mechanical, thermal, and chemical) and the dynamic or static nature of stimuli that provoke it. Usually the evoked pain stops after cessation of the stimulation, but sometimes it can persist for minutes, hours or even days, causing aftersensations. This aspect is mainly explained by involvement of a central sensitization process.

Paresthesia (an abnormal, non-painful sensation) and disesthesia (an abnormal, unpleasant and non-painful sensation) whether spontaneous or evoked, may coexist with pain. They can be described as crawling, numbness, itching and tingling sensations and reflect peripheral nociceptor hyperexcitability with spontaneous activity in low-threshold A-β afferents and respectively in C/A-δ afferents. (see table 2) (Baron et al., 2010).

Usually the screening tools provide immediate information and some of them can be fully applied to the patient without any prior physical examination, for example in the waiting room. Many of them are suitable to be used by the non-specialist physician in order to identify potential patients with neuropathic pain. However, these screening tools may miss 10-20% of patients with clinical diagnosed neuropathic pain. (Benett et al., 2007). There are many screening tools designed for the diagnosis and assessment of neuropathic pain and none of them cover the entire spectrum of symptoms and signs that might be encountered in this condition. It is possible, therefore, to use a combination of these questionnaires (see table 3) to get a good picture of neuropathic pain condition for an individual patient. (Cruccu et al., 2009)

### 2.2 Assessment of comorbidities

Comorbidities are recognized as a major factor that impact the outcome of neuropathic pain conditions. The most common spectrum of associated disorders includes poor quality of sleep, depression and anxiety.

| Symptoms/Questionnaire | LANSS | NPQ | DN4 | ID-Pain | painDetect | NPSI | StEP |
|---|---|---|---|---|---|---|---|
| | | | | | | | |
| Self reporting symptoms | • | | • | • | • | • | • |
| Ongoing pain rating | | | | | • | • | • |
| Electric shocks or shooting | • | • | • | • | • | • | |
| Hot or burning | • | • | • | • | • | • | • |
| Painful cold or freezing pain | | • | • | | | | • |
| Pricking, tingling pins, needles(any dysesthesia) | • | • | • | • | • | • | • |
| Numbness | | • | • | • | • | • | |
| Itching | | | • | | | | • |
| Pain provoked by light touching | • | • | | • | • | • | |
| Pain provoked by mild pressure | | | | | • | | |
| Pain provoked by heat or cold | | | | | • | | |
| Pain provoked by changes in weather | | • | | | | | |
| Pain provoked by activity or body position | | | | | | | • |
| Temporal patterns | | | | | • | | • |
| Pain limited to joints | | | | • | | | |
| Location, superficial or deep | | | | | | | • |
| Topography | | | | • | • | | |
| Radiation of pain | | | | | • | | |
| Autonomic changes | | | | • | | | |
| Affect disturbances | | • | | | | | |
| Physical examination | | | | | | | |
| Abnormal response to cold temperature (decrease or allodynia) | | | | | | | • |
| Hyperalgesia | | | | | | | • |
| Abnormal response to blunt pressure (decreased or evoked pain) | | | | | | | • |
| Decreased response to vibration | | | | | | | • |
| Brush allodynia | • | | • | | | | • |
| Raised soft touch threshold | | | • | | | | • |
| Raised pinprick threshold | • | | • | | | | • |
| Straight-leg-raising test | | | | | | | • |
| Skin changes | | | | | | | • |

Table 3. Screening tools-items inventory (modified from Bennett M.I. et al., 2007)

Patients who suffer from chronic pain experience difficulties in initiating and maintaining sleep. Sleep deprivation has been associated with a decreased pain threshold. The interrelationship of these factors is complex. Many chronic pain patients are depressed and anxious; sleep deprivation can lead to anxiety; and depression can be both the cause and the result of sleep disturbances. Therefore, sleep as well as mood should be evaluated in patients suffering from painful conditions. Several specific instruments are used in practice to elicit qualitative and quantitative information from chronic pain patients.

PHQ-9 and MOS sleep questionnaire were used to track co-morbidities in a study that assessed the PainDETECT questionnaire as a screening tool to predict the likelihood of a neuropathic pain component in chronic pain disorders (Lowe et al., 2004; Hays & Stewart, 1992).

The study revealed fundamental differences, in respect of perceived pain and of various co-morbidities, between low back pain patients with neuropathic and those with nociceptive components and provided important information on the association between neuropathic pain and the occurrence and severity of co-morbidities. Patients with neuropathic pain generally experience a more severe burden of co-morbid disorders than patients affected only by nociceptive type of pain (Freynhagen et al., 2006).

## 2.3 Neurological examination

An injury anywhere in the somatosensory system typically, leads to an area of sensory deficit distributed in the related innervations territory. These negative sensory signs may be expressed as a deficit in the mechanical or vibratory perception, which indicates damage of the large diameter afferent fibers or of the dorsal column tract. The picture could include also a deficit of noxious and thermal perception, which indicates damage of the small diameter afferent fibers or of the central pain processing pathways such as the spinothalamic tract.

A standardized bedside examination of patients with neuropathic pain must include the following components: touch, pressure, vibration, pinprick, cold, heat, temporal summation. The responses should be graded as normal, decreased or increased. When present, allodynia and hyperalgesia should be quantified by measuring the intensity and the area that is affected. It is generally agreed that assessment should be carried out in the area of maximum pain with the controlateral or neighboring reference area, free of pain, as a control if possible. Touch can be assessed by gently applying cotton swab or von Frey filaments of 2 g and 26 g strength to the skin, pin-prick sensation by the response to sharp pinprick stimuli, cold and heat sensation by measuring the response to thermal stimuli (e.g. metal objects kept at 20° C or 40° C), vibration sensation by the response to a tuning fork. (Arning & Baron, 2009)

Mechanical dynamic allodynia and mechanical static hyperalgesia can be evaluated using a painter's brush and respectively a blunt eraser end of a pencil. Abnormal temporal summation consists to increasing pain sensation (wind-up-like pain) from repetitive application of identical single noxious stimulus (mechanical or thermal) and is the clinical equivalent of increasing neuronal activity after repetitive noxious C-fiber stimulation of more than 3 Hz. The antagonists of NMDA receptors can block this process.

Inspection of the skin within the painful area is also an important gesture to note the presence of vasomotor, sweating and trophic changes which define sympathetic maintained pain and express a pathological adrenergic coupling between sympathetic postganglionic fibers and nociceptive afferent fibers.

In the chronic conditions, trophic changes of the skin and nails occur as do motor symptoms such as weakness, tremor and dystonia (Cruccu et al. 2004, Cruccu et al.,2009).

Nerve percussion at points of entrapment, compression or irritation can elicit electrical sensations, pins and needles in innervation's territory (Tinel's sign).

As in the case of spontaneous pain assessment, it is important to establish topographical distribution of evoked pains because as the neuroplastic changes develop, the pain distribution will no longer respect nerves, roots, segmental, cortical territory. Hence, primary hyperalgesia or allodynia represent pain provoked by stimuli applied within a nerve/root territory with ectopic activity. Secondary hyperalgesia or allodynia represents pain occurred by application of stimuli in the neighboring area of innervations territory of the injured nerve/root.

Neurological assessment of neuropathic pain also should include an examination of the autonomic nervous system and a detailed inventory of the somatomotor involvement to define the underlying disease and the extension of it. The distribution of the motor deficit could help us sometimes to differentiate between primary and secondary hyperalgesia/allodynia and to localize the injury.

As peripheral and central sensitization develop, in attempt to control pain, the harmful condition is most of the times no longer important because the neuropathic pain persists long after the cessation of the initial injury. However, the management of the ongoing underlying diseases (eg metabolic disorders) remains important rather to prevent appearance of new lesions of somatosensory nervous system than to control neuropathic pain (Baron et al., 2010).

However, the non-sensory neurologic symptoms and signs can independently contribute to pain and disability. In the case of associated weakness, patients are more prone to adopt vicious positions and therefore, mixed pain could develop by superimposing the nociceptive component related to joints or tendon structures (Dworkin et al. 2003).

### 2.4 Ancillary tests

When pain is the only manifestation of an injury in the somatosensory system, additional diagnostic information could come from the use of ancillary tests (see table 4).

Some aspects must be considered an attempt to use complementary tests to support the diagnosis and characterize the involvement of specific neuropathic pain mechanisms (Horowitz et al, 2007):

- using these laboratory tests, the presence, distribution and mechanisms of neuropathic pain only can be inferred because the available tests evaluate nervous system structures and functions presumed to be relevant to pain perception and transmission;
- since pain mediating fibers (small myelinated, Aδ, and unmyelinated, C fibers) are also responsible for other measurable functions, (e.g. temperature perception and autonomic

activity), many tests have focused on proving alterations in these modalities in order to verify A-δ or C-fiber damage;

- in the clinical expression of each particular disorder is a spectrum of symptoms and signs that reflect neural injury, with chronic pain occurring in only a small percentage of affected individuals.

| Fibers | Sensation | Testing | | | |
|---|---|---|---|---|---|
| | | Clinical | | Laboratory | |
| | | Bedside assessment | Expected pathological response | QST | Other |
| A-β | Touch | Piece of painter's brush or cotton swab | Reduced perception (hypoesthesia) | Von Frey filaments | NCS, SEPs |
| | Vibration | Tuning fork (128 Hz) | Reduced perception of threshold (pall-hypoesthesia) | Vibrameter | NCS, SEPs |
| A-δ | Pinprick, sharp pain | Prick skin with a pin single stimulus | Reduced perception (hypoalgesia) | Weighted needles | LEPs, IENF |
| | Cold | Thermoroller (20° C) | Reduced perception (thermal hypoesthesia) | Thermode | None |
| C | Warmth | Thermoroller (40° C) | Reduced perception (thermal hypoesthesia) | Thermode | LEPs, IENF |
| | Burning | none | - | Thermode | LEPs, IENF |

IENF intra-epidermal nerve fibre, LEP laser-evoked potential, NCS nerve conduction study, QST quantitative sensory testing: SEP, somatosensory-evoked potential

Table 4. Summary of assessment methods of nerve sensory functions (modified from Cruccu et al., 2004).

### 2.4.1 Clinical neurophysiology

The usual neurophysiologic tests (with surface electrodes for nerve stimulation and evoked potential recording) asses activity of the largest and fastest conducting sensory and motor myelinated nerve fibers (Aαβ). In order to assess the involvement of the central nervous system or the proximal part of the peripheral nerves, somatosensory and magnetic evoked potential studies can be helpful.

Although, unfortunately A-and C-fiber activities cannot be tested with these techniques, the abnormalities from these tests can be used to corroborate the clinical impression of damage to a specific peripheral nerve or to peripheral nerves in general as in a polyneuropathy (level A recommendation in the EFNS guidelines for neuropathic pain assessment, Cruccu et al., 2004).

### 2.4.2 Quantitative sensory testing

Quantitative sensory testing (QST) measures sensory thresholds for pain, touch, vibration and hot and cold temperature sensations. With this technology, specific fibers functions can be assessed: Aδ-fibers with cold and cold-pain detection thresholds, C-fibers with heat and heat-pain detection thresholds and large fiber (Aαβ) functions with vibration detection thresholds. The abnormal findings exist in both peripheral and central nervous disorder, without any distinction (Rolke et al., 2006).

It must be stressed that QST is a psychophysical test and therefore is highly dependent on the patient's alertness, concentration and motivation (level B recommendation EFNS guidelines for neuropathic pain assessment, Cruccu et al., 2004). QST is helpful to quantify the effects of treatments on allodynia and hyperalgesia and may reveal a different effect of treatments on different pain components (level A recommendation in the EFNS guidelines for neuropathic pain assessment, Cruccu et al., 2010).

### 2.4.3 Autonomic function testing

Autonomic evaluation is an important step in refining the neuropathic pain diagnosis based on the frequent association between neuropathic pain disorders and signs of autonomic dysfunction (dry eyes or mouth, changes in the color of the skin, temperature, sweating abnormalities, edema, orthostatic hypotension, etc) as well as the anatomic similarities between fibers processing pain and autonomic functions. The most useful tests are quantitative sudomotor axon reflex test (QSART), thermoregulatory sweat test, heart rate responses to deep breathing, Valsalva ratio, and surface skin temperature (Novak et al., 2001). The value of autonomic testing in patients with general neuropathic pain disorder, painful small-fiber neuropathy with burning feet has been shown in several studies. Autonomic abnormalities were seen in more than 90% of patients (Low et al, 2006).

### 2.4.4 Skin biopsy

In the recent years the histological study of unmyelinated nerve fibers in the skin had proved its utility by providing reliable diagnostic information when there is little or no clinical evidence of neuropathy, such as in a patient complaining of burning feet and to distinguish conditions mimicking a neuropathy. Epidermal nerve fiber density and morphology, complex ramifications, clustering, and axon swelling can be quantified (Devigli et al, 2003; Kennedy, 2004)

Reduced epidermal innervations density has been used as mandatory criteria for the diagnosis of a small fiber neuropathy (level B recommendation in the EFNS guideline of neuropathic pain assessment, Cruccu et al., 2004, 2009).

### 2.4.5 Laser evoked potential

Laser evoked potential (LEP) based on radiant-heat pulse stimuli delivered by laser stimulators, provide a selective activation of the afferent fibers and the free nerve endings (A-δ and C) (Bromm et al. 1984). The cortical networks that generate LEPs are able to detect abrupt changes in the sensory input, but are much less qualified to reflect a slow-changing state. Thus, LEPs are inappropriate to reflect the slowly emerging, ill-defined and long lasting phenomena that underlie over-reaction symptoms (hyperalgesia and allodynia), which are thought to depend on spino-reticulo-thalamic projection system . Late LEPs reflect activity of the A-fibers and ultralate LEPs of the unmyelinated nociceptive pathways (Garcia-Larrea & Godinho, 2007).

For the purpose of studying peripheral and central neuropathic pain, LEP are the most sensitive tool compared with any other neurophysiologic test. The finding of a LEP suppression helps to diagnose neuropathic pain (level A recommendation in the EFNS guideline neuropathic pain assessment, Cruccu et al., 2009).

### 2.5 Pathophysiology – From symptoms and signs to mechanism and vice versa

Our ability to translate pain complaints and sensory signs into specific physiopathologic mechanisms which will have implications for appropriate therapy is only in the beginnings (Baron et al. 2010). However, all this process of translation is difficult because:

- one single mechanism can give rise to several different symptoms; the same mechanism can be found in various diseases;
- in one individual patient different mechanisms might be involved;
- many of these mechanisms are independent on the etiology of a particular disorder;
- different mechanisms could lead to the same symptom or sign.

Different treatment regimens are needed for different pain mechanisms, thereby a mechanism based treatment approach would result in efficient analgesia. Hence, to progress at this point we have to assume that pain mechanisms can be identified by analyzing patient's individual symptoms and signs (see table 5).

At present, there are some data that could help us to understand the associations between at least some symptoms and suggested underlying mechanisms (Jensen & Baron, 2003).

It is worth to mention that the pain system is not static and the changes occur in a dynamic, step-up, from periphery to central and somewhat unpredictable manner whenever the system is activated (Baron, 2006).

A useful, oversimplified approach is to differentiate processes that involve the following (Finnerup &Jensen, 2006):

- increased firing in primary afferent nociceptors (e.g. ectopic discharges as a result of abnormal redistribution of sodium channels in damaged peripheral nerve fibers)
- changes in the central processing of sensory signals (central sensitization) and, consequently, normal sensory perception is amplified and sustained;
- decreased inhibition of neuronal activity in the central structures (e.g due to loss of inhibitory neurons)

#### 2.5.1 Ectopic nerve activity

Ectopic nerve activity has been involved in many *positive phenomena* (spontaneous, ongoing or paroxysmal pain, primary hyperalgezia/allodynia), characteristic of neuropathic pain:

- *ongoing spontaneous pain* and *paroxysmal stimulus-independent pain* has been correlated with ectopic impulse generation within the nociceptive pathways, either within nociceptive afferent fibers (C- and Aδ-fibers), either in the dorsal root ganglion or at the level of the second-order nociceptive neuron by increasing expression of voltage-gated sodium channels and secondary lowering action potential threshold until ectopic activity takes place (Amir et al. 2005; Wu et al., 2002)

| Mechanism | Symptoms | Targets |
|---|---|---|
| **Peripheral nociceptor hyperexcitability** | | |
| Ectopic impulses generation, oscillations in dorsal root ganglion | Paroxysmal shooting spontaneous pain | Sodium channels |
| **Peripheral nociceptor sensitization** | | |
| Inflammation within nerves: cytokine release | Ongoing spontaneous pain | Cytokines |
| Reduced activation threshold to: | | |
| Heat | Heat allodynia | TRPV1 receptor |
| Cold | Cold allodynia | TRPM8 receptor |
| Mechanical stimuli | Static mechanical allodynia | ASCI receptor(?) |
| Noradrenaline | Sympathetic maintained pain | α receptor |
| **Central dorsal horn hyperexcitability** | | |
| Central sensitization on spinal level<br>Ongoing C-input induces increased synaptic transmission | | |
| Amplification of C fibers input | Ongoing spontaneous pain | Presynaptic:<br>-μ-receptors<br>-calcium channels(α2-δ)<br>Postsynaptic:<br>-NMDA receptors<br>-sodium channels<br>-NK1 receptors |
| Gating of Aβ- fibers input | Mechanical dynamic allodynia | |
| Gating of Aδ- fibers input | Mechanical static hyperalgesia | |
| Reduction intraspinal inhibitory interneurons | | |
| GABA-ergic | Ongoing spontaneous pain<br>Evoked pain | GABA-B receptors |
| Opiodergic | Ongoing spontaneous pain<br>Evoked pain | μ-receptors |
| Changes in supraspinal descending modulation | | |
| Decreased inhibitory control (NA, 5-HT) | Ongoing spontaneous pain<br>Evoked pain | α2 receptor<br>5-HT receptors |
| Increased faciliatory control | Ongoing spontaneous pain<br>Evoked pain | |

Table 5. Mechanisms-symptoms correlations (modified from Baron R. et al., 2006)

- *heat hyperalgezia* in addition to ongoing burning pain can have as underlying mechanism spontaneous nerve activity induced by changing expression of vanilloid receptor (TRPV1, physiologically activated by noxious heat at about 41°C, and additional sensitization to heat by intracellular signal transduction (Fischer & Reeh, 2007). After a nerve lesion TRPV1 is downregulated on injured nerve fibers and upregulated on uninjured C-fibers (Caterina & Julius, 2001).
- abnormal function and expression of TRPM8, a cold sensitive receptor of TRP family, triggered by nerve lesion, with secondary ongoing ectopic discharges have been recently identified in a patient with painful neuropathy in combination with *cold allodynia* (Serra et al., 2009).

### 2.5.2 Central sensitisation

Central sensitization can manifest in three ways ((Woolf, 1992; Jensen & Baron, 2003):

- enlargement of the peripheral area where a stimulus will determine neuronal activation (secondary hyperalgezia/ allodynia);
- increased response to suprathreshold input (hyperalgezia, hyperpatia)
- previously subthreshold input reach threshold and initiate action potential discharge ( allodynia, in particular dynamic mechanical allodynia).

Central sensitization might develop as a consequence of ectopic activity in the primary nociceptive afferent fibers without any structural damage within the central nervous system. Ongoing discharges of peripheral afferent fibers lead to postsynaptic changes of the second-order nociceptive neurons, such as phosphorylation of NMDA and AMPA receptors (Ultenius et al., 2007) or expression of voltage-gated sodium channels (Lai et al., 2003).These changes determine neuronal hyperexcitability that allow the mechanosensitive Aβ and Aδ afferent fibers with low-threshold to activate second-order nociceptive neurons. As a consequence, normally innocuous tactile stimuli such as light brushing or pricking the skin become painful. This phenomena are called dynamic and punctate mechanical allodynia (Hains et al, 2004).

### 2.5.3 Decreased inhibition of neuronal activity in the central nervous structures

After a peripheral nerve lesion there is a loss of inhibitory GABAergic interneurons in the spinal horn. Prevention of interneurons cell death attenuates mechanical and thermal hyperalgesia, indicating that desinhibition contributes to neuropathic pain (Moore et al., 2002). There are, also, other inhibitory neurons, such as descending pathways originating in the brainstem, which contribute to modulation of pain and any injury of these opioidergic and monoaminergic systems lead to pain exacerbation via a disinhibition process. Paroxysms are traditionally thought to be generated by ectopic ongoing discharges from sodium channels and, therefore, may respond to sodium-channel blockers (Black et al., 2008; Siqueira et al., 2009). However, paroxysms can, also, be seen in patients with small fiber neuropathy and deafferentation, pointing to a central mechanism and are reported to be relieved by tricyclic antidepressants and serotonin-noradrenaline reuptake inhibitors, suggesting changes in supraspinal descending modulation with decreasing monoaminergic inhibitory control (Jensen & Baron, 2003).

### 2.5.4 Attempts to group patients according to sensory profiles

The complexity of neuropathic pain pathophysiology and translating process from mechanisms to symptoms and signs, suggests that the individual pattern of sensory abnormalities most likely closely reflects the underlying pain-generating mechanism (Baron, 2010). To identify phenotypic subgroups of patients with distinct sensory pattern several approaches were used:

- a standardized psychophysical technique to test both the nociceptive and non-nociceptive afferent systems (QST- quantitative sensory testing) was recently proposed by the German Network on Neuropathic Pain(DFNS). The DFNS nationwide multicentre trial comprised complete sensory profiles of 1236 patients with different types of neuropathic pain. The study conclusion was that a certain association of symptoms and signs could suggest a particular underlying mechanisms. For example, a combination of heat hyperalgesia with mechanical allodynia and mechanical hyperalgesia could indicate peripheral ectopic activity at the level of heat sensitive nociceptors that triggers a process of central sensitization. On the other hand, in patients with complete sensory loss is very unlikely that peripheral mechanisms are responsible for maintaining neuropathic pain (Meier et al., 2010).
- in another study the tool used to identify relevant subgroups of patients with postherpetic neuralgia and painful diabetic neuropathy who were characterized by a specific symptom profile, was the pain symptom questionnaire. Using a hierarchical cluster analysis were determined five distinct subgroups of patients. The sensory profiles showed remarkable differences in the expression of the symptoms, all subgroups occurring in both diseases but with different frequencies (Baron et al., 2009).
- In one study the neuropathic symptoms and sings were assessed using a structured interview and standardized bedside examination in patients with painful diabetic neuropathy, postherpetic neuralgia and radicular back pain as well as in a group of patients with non-neuropathic pain. The physical examination was considered more important for the distinction of pain subtypes than were the assessment of symptoms during the interview (Woolf et al., 1998).

All these different techniques to identify subgroups of patients show that there are phenotypic differences based on certain combinations of sensory abnormalities across the different etiologies and neuropathic pain syndromes. These efforts to identify and understand the underlying mechanisms involved in neuropathic pain will lead us to a more effective and specific mechanism based treatment approach. However, the management of neuropathic pain is, also, a matter of timing. The distinction between peripheral and central sensitization could be critical in the evolution and appropriate treatment of neuropathic pain (Attal et al., 2008; Baron et al., 2010).

## 2.6 Neuropathic pain diagnosis in special populations

### 2.6.1 Neuropathic pain in children

Most of the common neuropathic pain syndromes seen in adults are rare in pediatric population and some others are not even encountered. For example neuropathic pain from diabetic polineuropathy is never a significant concern in children. Pain as a consequence of stroke or radiculopathy or trigeminal neuralgia is tremendously rare in this period of life.

Children with plexus avulsion at birth or traumatic nerve injuries rarely develop neuropathic pain as most of the adult population does in a similar context. Also some conditions gain increasing recognition in this special group.The spectrum of etiologies that induce neuropathic pain in children are mostly related to trauma, postsurgery, infectious myelitides, neuropathies (autoimmune, genetic), complex regional pain syndrome or phantom limb. Some of the rare neuropathic pain syndromes are exclusively encountered at this age: mitochondrial disorders, eritromelalgia, Fabry disease, lead intoxication (Walco et al. 2010).

Favorable neuroplasticity in younger patients might be the cause of a better recovery with lower incidence for neuropathic pain comparing to adults. Tools used in evaluation of adults with neuropathic pain could be extrapolated in children but aspects related to the developmental process should always taken into account as potentially modifiers of clinical expression. The assessment of pain and somatosensory examination is a challenging step in children. Appropriate instruments adapted for pediatric population are only developed for other types of pain: musculoskeletal, abdominal or headache (Craig & Korol, 2008).

A controlled study conducted in a group of children aged 7 to 17 with unilateral CRPS using QST showed that patients displayed cold allodinia and a combination of dynamic mechanical allodinia and hyperalgezia to pinprick (Tan et al., 2008).

A study that compared from medical records adult patients and children with CRPS and concluded that the skin temperature at onset was cooler among children, the lower extremity was involved more frequently and presence of sympathetic symptoms and abnormal neurological signs and symptoms were milder (Sethna et al., 2007).

### 2.6.2 Neuropathic pain in the elderly

Prevalence of neuropathic pain in the elderly population over 65 years of age is estimated around 9%(Bouhassira et al., 2007).

Different etiologies may be responsible for neuropathic painful condition in older people but the most frequent are related to diabetes, shingles, radiculopathies and stroke. Most of the people in this group of age do not report pain adequately and usually think that pain is a normal part of the aging process (Pickering & Capriz, 2008).

The most challenging points regarding the diagnostic approach in this age group are related to cognitive impairment and high incidence of affective disorders that will impact the way people report their pain or collaborate in answering to sometimes difficult questionnaires. Also comorbities are usually accumulated in this population and the chance of facing different types of pain (joints inflammation, visceral, neoplastic, related to treatments) is considerably high (Weiner et al., 2006).

Instruments of pain assessment should be appropriate with the patient cognitive status and medical personnel should observe the patient's behavior. Best instruments are the numeric and visual scale but also faces and behavioral scales (Pickering, 2005).

### 2.6.3 Lessons learnt from randomized clinical trials (RCT's) for neuropathic pain

Most of the clinical trials were addressed to neuropathic pain associated with herpes zoster infection or diabetic neuropathy.

Regarding the outcome of different therapies, realistic expectations are defined by at least 30 % of pain alleviation. Multiple dimensions of pain experience need to take into consideration sleep quality, depression and social impact. As a consequence, the efficacy of a certain therapy must be judged also from this perspective (Moulin et al., 2007).

Evidences showed that different mechanisms and sensory profiles might be encountered in painful conditions with a similar etiology and conversely, one mechanism or sensory profile could be associated with different etiologies. For example cold hyperalgesia could be present in traumatic nerve injury but also in central post-stroke pain. Sympatheticaly maintained pain might characterize CRPS but also the acute pain in herpes zoster infection. As the time passes after the initial injury, multiple mechanisms get involved and become responsible for painful symptoms (Baron, 2006)

Based on this observation, trials that used drugs combination as opioids and calcium channel ligands reported a better outcome with lower doses compared with single drug administration (Gilron et al., 2005, Hanna et al., 2008). Caution is recommended for combining tricyclic antidepressants and tramadol regarding the risk of "serotonine syndrome".

The major classes of medication used for pharmacological treatment of neuropathic pain have different modes of action. Sometimes is difficult to understand how the specific mode of action of a certain drug interfere with the painful symptoms explained by a particular mechanism. On the other hand the success of a certain therapeutic intervention in alleviating pain is a clear opportunity to test a hypothesis regarding a certain association between mechanism and symptoms (Dworkin et al., 2003)

Tricyclic antidepressants act on monoamine reuptake, also block sodium channels and have anticholinergic effects as well. Apart from improving depression and sleep, this class of medication has unquestionable analgesic effect. Therefore is rated as level A indication for diabetic polineuropathy and postherpectic neuralgia and level B for central pain and chronic radiculopathy.

Serotonine end norepinephrine selective reuptake inhibitors are only studied in diabetic polyneuropathies and rated level A for evidence of efficacy. No other relevant information is available regarding their action in other painful conditions.

Calcium channel ligands lead to decrease of neurotransmitter release by acting on central terminals of primary nociceptive neurons were widely tested in the traditional models (DPN and PHN) but also in central pain syndromes and cancer related painful conditions.

Similarly the agonists of opioid receptors demonstrated efficacy in several RCT's conducted for peripheral as well as central neuropathic pain syndromes, cancer related and phantom pain (Dworkin et al., 2007).

Topical application of lidocaine was demonstrated to be efficient in a patient population characterized by peripheral localized pain and allodynia as occurs in PHN. Its action is explained by a nonspecific blockage of sodium channels in the peripheral afferent fibers. Although patients displaying allodynia are considered the best candidates and represented the majority in clinical trials, patients without allodynia might have considerable benefit as well (Baron et al., 2009b).

Single dose capsaicin patch (8%) apart from excellent results in PHN trials (Backonja et al., 2008), also proved it's efficacy in treating pain related to HIV infection where other drugs had negative results (pregabaline, amytriptiline and topical lidocaine). Capsaicin patch acts as an agonist of TRPV1 receptor expressed on nociceptive nerve fibers in the skin (Simpson et al., 2008).

The complex psychosocial aspects of neuropathic pain are sometimes addressed only by an integrated multidisciplinary approach including pharmacological and non-pharmacologic treatment strategies such as cognitive, behavioral, physical and occupational therapy (Oerlemans et al., 2000). For example an original concept such as graded motor imagery (mirror therapy) has been demonstrated to be efficient in reducing pain in patients suffering from CRPS or phantom pain (Moseley, 2006; Ramachandran & Altschuler, 2009).

Interventional therapy is indicated for patients who failed to obtain sufficient relief with standard medication. RCT's showed efficacy for invasive interventions in drug resistant patients with failed back surgery syndrome, postherpetic neuralgia or CRPS. Studies using functional magnetic resonance imaging (fMRI) in patients under spinal cord stimulation (SCS) found increased activation of the medial primary sensorimotor cortex, contralateral posterior insula, and the ipsilateral secondary somatosensory cortex (S2). Decreased activation was seen in the bilateral primary motor cortices and the ipsilateral primary somatosensory cortex (Stančák et al., 2009)

## 3. Case discussions

### 3.1 Case 1

Male of 65 years old, known with myasthenia gravis under prednisone as immunosuppressive treatment developed herpes zoster infection in the left C3, C4, and C5 roots territory. He reported pain starting after 10 days from the vesicular rash onset and respecting the same distribution. During the first interview (3 months distance after vesicular rash remision) he described pain as a superficial burning, hot wire or shooting. Also he felt his skin like as a "cardboard". His pain was coming and going in episodes that lasted seconds with complete pain free periods between these episodes. The intensity was rated 10 on the numeric rating scale and the daily activity and sleep were significantly disturbed. He had itching, pain attacks like electric shocks and very slight sensation of numbness in the painful area. The light touching, slight pressure and warm water elicited pain. The neurological exam showed an increased threshold to pinprick sensation, static and dynamic mechanical allodynia, heat allodynia and temporal summation in the painful area. On the skin, small areas of abnormal paleness have been noted as a consequence of rash healing (figure 1a, b). We used for assessment of pain, painDetect questionnaire and StEP. The total score obtained for painDetect was 21 and was considered positive for neuropathic pain.

The paroxysmal pain, dysesthesia, raised pinprick threshold and threshold decreased for noxious heat stimuli pointed to a partial deafferentation of C and some of Aδ fibers and spontaneous activity in nociceptive afferents, probably related to abnormal expression of voltage-gated sodium channels and vanilloid receptor, TRPV1. The clinical picture also suggests central sensitization process on spinal level by pre- and post-synaptic changes on second-order neuron induced by ongoing C input: temporal summation, mechanical dynamic and static allodynia. Analyzing the patient's pain in this manner, it is easier to choose the potential optimal pharmacological agents. For this patient a selective sodium channel blocker, like carbamazepine or tricyclic antidepressive and μ-receptors agonists, opioids, are not suitable because of myasthenia gravis. A calcium-channel blocker α2-δ ligand was recommended with a rating of 8 (VAS) for the mean pain intensity per month. Further local application of capsaicin patch (8%) lowered the pain up to a rating of 5, which the patient considered acceptable in the long run.

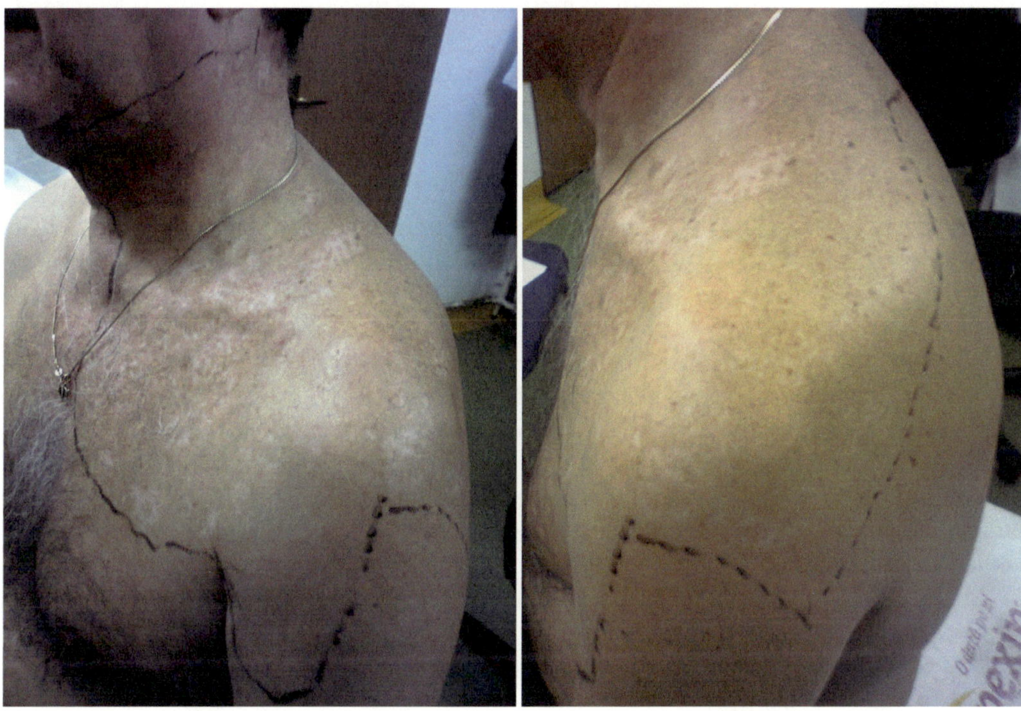

Fig. 1. a) Fig. 1. b)

Fig. 1.

### 3.2 Case 2

Male of 47 years old was operated for lumbar disc herniation at L4-L5 manifested as acute severe low back pain associated with diffusely distributed and intermittent left leg pain in the groin and anterior thigh and a part of the lower leg. Postoperatively, a novel pain has occurred immediately after surgery. The patient was examined at 6 months interval from onset.This time the pain has been spontaneous, permanent, with a clear distribution in left

L5 root territory (left lateral lower leg and medial dorsum of foot toward the big toe). The pain's intensity was rated 8/10 on the numeric rating scale, and the words sharp, stabbing, squeezing were used as descriptors. Also, the light touch on the dorsum of the foot determines pain. The low back pain still persists but only related to movements. No negative signs were found at the neurological exam.

Compared to the pain before surgery, the actual pain has a specific topography for L5 root territory and it could be considered as a neuropathic one, even if the specific pain descriptors were missing. The pain is generated in the spinal root and not in the painful area. Mechanical dynamic allodynia described, is the expression of central sensitization. In this case, the central sensitization did not occurr secondary to ongoing C fibers input, instead of that, gating of Aβ-fiber input, reduction of intraspinal inhibitory interneurons and changes in supraspinal descending modulation are the most probable mechanisms to explain the patient's pain. Based on this judgment, topical pharmacological agents are useless. NMDA-receptor antagonists, μ-receptor agonists, GABA-B agonists or spinal cord stimulation are the reasonable options.

### 3.3 Case 3

Male of 45 years old complained about painful legs and weakness since he had an acute motor-sensory axonal neuropathy (AMSAN). The intensity of pain has been 9 from ten points on the numeric rating scale. The patient has spontaneous pain attacks superimposed on a milder but permanent pain largely distributed over the distal part of the limbs, but predominantly in the lower limbs where pain usually rise up to the knees. The words used to describe pain are: burning, electric shocks and stabbing. Also,at the interview he complained that the pain could be provoked by light touch, slight pressure and heat and also reports an abnormal sensation such as prickling and numbness. The total score on painDetect questionnaire was 27, which is positive for neuropathic character of pain. Clinical examination revealed symmetrical weakness in all limbs, more in the legs, mechanical dynamic and static allodynia, heat allodynia, raised threshold to heat stimuli but the skin looked permanent cold and cyanotic skin and sometimes swollen and reddish when the pain was more intense. The clinical picture present many elements which suggest peripheral sensitization (dysesthesia, heat allodynia and raised threshold to heat) associated with abnormal recruiting of sympathetic nervous system. The central sensitization is pointed by mechanical dynamic and static allodynia. In this case because of the presence of sympathetic maintained pain, it seems logical to recommend tricyclic antidepressive drugs or sympathetic block, but it will not be sufficient and combination with other kind of drugs (calcium channel blocker, α2-δ ligands, μ-receptor agonists, NMDA receptors antagonists) will be of very much help .

## 4. Conclusion

The effort of grouping patients according to sensory profiles will allow us to better understand the mechanisms involved in neuropathic pain development and persistence. Future trials will probably select specific sensory profiles across different etiologies and test treatment interventions from other perspectives.

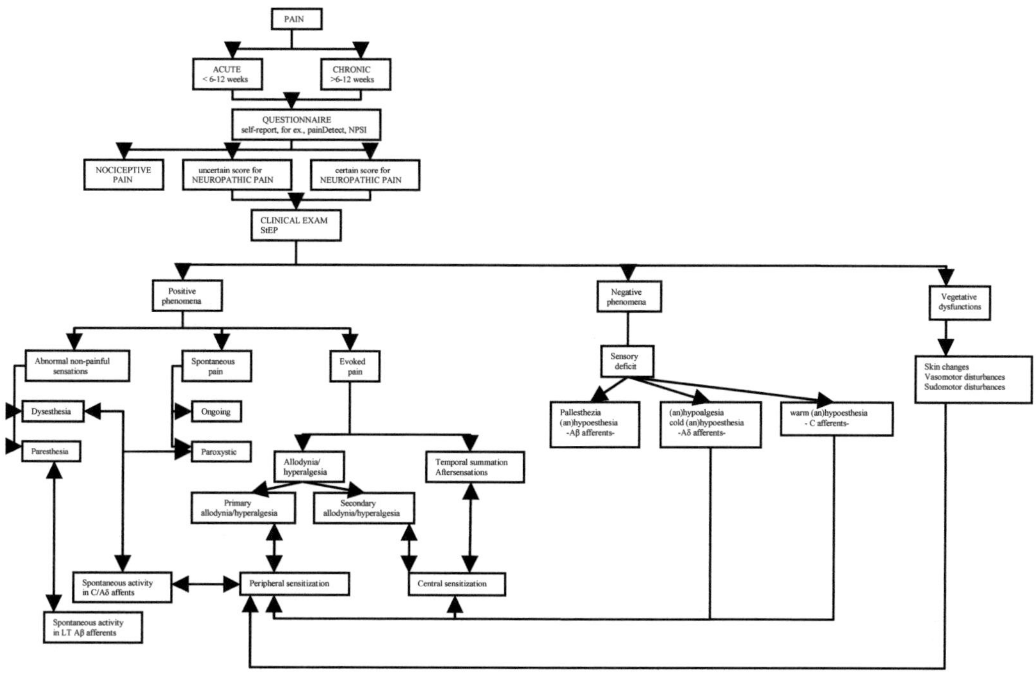


Fig. 2. Proposed algorithm for systematic approach for neuropathic pain assessment

## 5. References


[1] Amir R, Kocsis JD, Devor M.(2005). Multiple interacting sites of ectopic spike electrogenesis in primary sensory neurons. *J Neurosci*; 25: 2576–85. ISSN:0270-6474

[2] Arning K, Baron R. (2009). Evaluation of symptom heterogeneity in neuropathic pain using assessments of sensory functions. *Neurotherapeutics*; 6: 738–48. ISSN: 1933-7213

[3] Attal N, Fermanian C, Fermanian J, Lanteri-Minet M, Alchaar H, Bouhassira D. (2008). Neuropathic pain: are there distinct subtypes depending on the aetiology or anatomical lesion? *Pain.*;138(2):343-353. ISSN: 0304-3959

[4] Backonja M, Wallace MS, Blonsky ER. (2008). NGX-4010, a high concentration capsaicin patch, for the treatment of postherpetic neuralgia: a randomised, double-blind study. *Lancet Neurol*; 7: 1106–12. ISSN: 1474-4422

[5] Baron R. (2006). Mechanism of Disease: neuropathic pain-a clinical perspective. *Nat. Clin. Pract. Neurol*; 2: 95–106. ISSN: 1745-834X

[6] Baron R, Tolle TR, Gockel U, Brosz M, Freynhagen R.( 2009). A crosssectional cohort survey in 2100 patients with painful diabetic neuropathy and postherpetic neuralgia: differences in demographic data and sensory symptoms, *Pain*; 146: 34–40. ISSN: 0304-3959

[7] Baron R, Mayoral V, Leijon G, Binder A, Steigerwald I, Serpell M. (2009) 5% lidocaine medicated plaster versus pregabalin in post-herpetic neuralgia and diabetic

polyneuropathy: an open-label, non- inferiority two-stage RCT study. *Curr Med Res Opin;* 25: 1663–76. ISSN: 0300-7995
[8] Baron R., Binder A., Wasner G.(2010).Neuropathic pain: diagnosis, pathophysiological mechanism and treatment. *Lancet Neurology*. 9:807-19. ISSN: 1474-4422
[9] Bennett MI, Attal N, Backonja MM. (2007). Using screening tools to identify neuropathic pain. *Pain*. 127: 199–203. ISSN: 0304-3959
[10] Bennett MI (2001) The LANSS Pain Scale: The Leeds Assessment of Neuropathic Symptoms and Signs. *Pain* 92: 147–157. ISSN: 0304-3959
[11] Black JA, Nikolajsen L, Kroner K, Jensen TS, Waxman SG. (2008). Multiple sodium channel isoforms and mitogen-activated protein kinases are present in painful human neuromas, *Ann Neurol;* 64: 644–53. ISSN: 0364-5134
[12] Boucsein C, Kettenmann H, Nolte C. (2000). Electrophysiological properties of microglial cells in normal and pathologic rat brain slices. *Eur J Neurosci*, 12:2049-2058. ISSN: 1460-9568
[13] Bouhassira D., Attal N., Fermanian J., Alchaar H., Gautron M., Masquelier E., Rostaing S., Lanteri-Minet M., Collin E., Grisare J., Boureau F. (2004). Development and validation of the Neuropathic Pain Symptom Inventory. *Pain* 108 248–257; ISSN: 0304-3959
[14] Bouhassira D, Attal N, Alchaar H, Boureau F, Bruxelle J, Cunin G, et al. (2005). Comparison of pain syndromes associated with nervous or somatic lesions and development of a new neuropathic pain diagnostic questionnaire (DN4). *Pain;*114:29–36. ISSN: 0304-3959
[15] Bouhassira D, Lantéri-Minet M, Attal N, Laurent B, Touboul C. (2008) Prevalence of chronic pain with neuropathic characteristics in the general population. *Pain* 136(3):380-7. ISSN: 0304-3959
[16] Bromm B, Treede RD. (1984). Nerve fibre discharges, cerebral potentials and sensations induced by CO2 laser stimulation, *Hum Neurobiol,* 3:33–40; ISSN: 0721-9075
[17] Caterina MJ, Julius D., (2001) The vanilloid receptor: a molecular gateway to the pain pathway, *Annu Rev Neurosci;* 24: 487–517. ISSN: 0147-006X
[18] Cruccu G.,. Anand P, Attal N., Garcia-Larrea L., Haanpää M., Jørum E.,. Serra J, and Jensen T. S. (2004) EFNS guidelines on neuropathic pain assessment, *European Journal of Neurology*, 11: 153–162; ISSN: 1351-5101
[19] Cruccu G., Truini A. (2009). Tools for Assessing Neuropathic Pain. *PLoS Med.*, doi: 10.1371/journal.pmed.1000045;
[20] Cruccu G., Sommera C., Anand P., N. Attal, Baron R., Garcia-Larrea L., Haanpa M.,. Jensen T. S, Serra J. and. Treede R.D., (2010) EFNS guidelines on neuropathic pain assessment: revised 2009. *European Journal of Neurology;* 17(8):1010-18. ISSN: 1351-5101
[21] Craig KD, Korol CT. (2008). Developmental issues in understanding, assessing, and managing pediatric pain. In: *Pain in Children: A Practical Guide for Primary Care*. Walco GA, Goldschneider KR, eds. Totowa, NJ 07512: Humana Press; 9-20. USA, ISBN:978-1-934115-31-2
[22] Devigili G., Tugnoli V., Penza P., Camozzi F., Lombardi R., Melli G., Broglio L., Granieri E., Lauria G.,(2003). The diagnostic criteria for small fibre neuropathy: from symptoms to neuropathology, *Brain;* 131:1912-1925. ISSN: 0006-8950

[23] Dworkin RH, Backonja M, Rowbotham MC, Allen RR, Argoff CR, Bennett GJ, Bushnell MC, Farrar JT, Galer BS, Haythornthwaite JA, Hewitt DJ, Loeser JD, Max MB, Saltarelli M, Schmader KE, Stein C, Thompson D, Turk DC, Wallace MS, Watkins LR, Weinstein SM. (2003).Advances in Neuropathic Pain: diagnosis, mechanism and treatment recommendations. *Arch Neurol.*;60(11):1524-1534. ISSN: 1013-3119

[24] Finnerup N., Troels J.S. , (2006). Mechanisms of Disease: mechanism-based classification of neuropathic pain—a critical analysis, *Nature Clinical Practice*;2(2)107-15. ISSN: 1745-834X

[25] Fischer MJ, Reeh PW.(2007). Sensitization to heat through G-proteincoupled receptor pathways in the isolated sciatic mouse nerve, *Eur J Neurosci*; 25: 3570–75. ISSN: 1351-5101

[26] Freynhagen R, Baron R, Gockel U, Tolle T., (2006). PainDetect: a new screeing questionnaire to detect neuropathic components in patients with back pain, *Curr Med Res Opin*;22: 1911–20. ISSN: 0300-7995

[27] Galer BS, Jensen MP. (1997). Development and preliminary validation of a pain measure specific to neuropathic pain: the Neuropathic Pain Scale., *Neurology*;48:332–8. ISSN:0028-3878

[28] Garcia-Larrea L., Godinho F., (2007). Diagnostic Role of Laser-evoked Potentials in Central Neuropathic Pain, *European neurological disease.II*

[29] Gilron I, Bailey JM, Tu D, Holden RR, Weaver DF, Houlden RL. Morphine, gabapentin, or their combination for neuropathic pain. (2005). *N Engl J Med*; 352: 1324–34.

[30] Gilron I., Peter C., Watson N., Cahill M., Moulin E. (2006).Neuropathic Pain: a practical guide for the clinician, CMAJ. ISSN: 0820-3946.

[31] Gosselin RD, Suter MR, Ji RR, Decosterd I (2010): Glial Cells and Chronic Pain. *Neuroscientist*. 16(5):519-31. ISSN:1073-8584.

[32] Gray P. (2008). Acute neuropathic pain: diagnosis and treatment, *Current Opinion in Anaesthesiology*.21(5):590-595. ISSN: 0952—7907.

[33] Haanpaa M., Attal N., Backonja M., Baron R., Bouhassira D., Crrucu G., Hansson P., Haithomthwaite JA, Iannetti GD, Jensen TS,, Kaupila T., Nurmikko TJ, Rice AS, RowbothamM., Serra J., Sommer C., Smith BH, Treede RD.(2011). NeuPSIG guidelines on neuropathic pain assessment. *Pain*. 152(1):14-27.ISSN: 0304-3959

[34] Hains BC, Saab CY, Klein JP, Craner MJ, Waxman SG. (2004).Altered sodium channel expression in second-order spinal sensory neurons contributes to pain after peripheral nerve injury., *J Neurosci*; 24: 4832–39. ISSN: 0270-6474

[35] Hanna M, O'Brien C, Wilson MC. (2008). Prolonged-release oxycodone enhances the effects of existing gabapentin therapy in painful diabetic neuropathy patients. *Eur J Pain*; 12: 804–13. ISSN: 1090-3801

[36] Hayes C, Browne S., Burstal R., (2002). Neuropathic pain in the acute pain service: a prospective survey, *Acute Pain*; 4;2; 45-8. ISSN: 1366-0071

[37] Jensen T. S., Towards a mechanism-based approach to the treatment of neuropathic pain. In: Neuropathic *Pain: Bench to Bedside* - International Congress and Symposium Series 259-2005;

[38] Jensen T. S., Baron R., (2003).Translation of symptoms and signs into mechanism in neuropathic pain,; *Pain*;102(1-2):1-8. ISSN: 0304-3959

[39] Ji RR, Suter MR. (2007). p38 MAPK, microglial signaling, and neuropathic pain. *Mol Pain*, 3:33. ISSN: 1744-8069.

[40] Kaki AM, El-Yaski AZ, Youseif E., (2005). Identifying neuropathic pain among patients with chronic low-back pain: use of the Leeds Assessment of Neuropathic Symptoms and Signs pain scale, *Reg Anesth Pain Med*; 30:422–8. ISSN: 1098-7339

[41] Karanikolas M., Aretha D., Tsolakis, I. et al., Optimized perioperative analgesia reduces chronic phantom limb pain intensity, prevalence, and frequency: a prospective, randomized, clinical trial, *Anesthesiology*, vol. 114, no. 5, pp. 1144–1154. ISSN: 003-3022

[42] Krause SJ, Backonja MM. (2003). Development of a Neuropathic Pain Questionnaire, *Clin J Pain*; 19:306–14. ISSN: 0749-8047.

[43] Kennedy WR., Opportunities afforded by the study of unmyelinated nerves in skin and other organs.(2004). *Muscle Nerve*; 29:756–67. ISSN: 0148-639X

[44] Kennedy WR,Wendelschafer-Crabb G, Polydefkis M, et al., Pathology and quantitation of cutaneous innervation. (2005) In: *Peripheral neuropathy*. Dyck PJ, Thomas PK, editors. 4th edition. Philadelphia (PA): Elsevier Saunders;. p. 869–95; USA

[45] Lai J, Hunter JC, Porreca F., (2003). The role of voltage-gated sodium channels in neuropathic pain, *Curr Opin Neurobiol*; 13: 291–97. ISSN: 0959-4388.

[46] Low VA, Sandroni P, Fealey RD, et al. (2006). Detection of small-fiber neuropathy by sudomotor testing, *Muscle Nerve*; 34:57–61. ISSN: 0148-639X.

[47] Ma W, Zhang Y, Bantel C, Eisenach JC. (2005). Medium and large injured dorsal root ganglion cells increase TRPV-1, accompanied by increased alpha2C-adrenoceptor co-expression and functional inhibition by clonidine. *Pain*; 113: 386–94. ISSN: 0304-3959.

[48] Maier C, Baron R, Toelle T, et al. (2010). Quantitative Sensory Testing in the German Research Network on Neuropathic Pain (DFNS): somatosensory abnormalities in 1236 patients with different neuropathic pain syndromes. *Pain*; 150(3):439-450. ISSN: 0304-3959.

[49] McGrath PJ, Walco GA, Turk DC, et al. PedIMMPACT. (2008). Core outcome domains and measures for pediatric acute and chronic/recurrent pain clinical trials: PedIMMPACT recommendations. *J Pain*. 9(9):771-783.

[50] Moore KA, Kohno T, Karchewski LA, Scholz J, Baba H, Woolf CJ. (2002). Partial peripheral nerve injury promotes a selective loss of GABAergic inhibition in the superficial dorsal horn of the spinal cord. *J Neurosci*; 22: 6724–31. ISSN: 0270-6474.

[51] Moseley GL. (2006). Graded motor imagery for pathologic pain: a randomized controlled trial. *Neurology*; 67: 2129–34. ISSN: 0028-3878

[52] Moulin DE, Clark AJ, Gilron I, et al. (2007). Pharmacological management of chronic neuropathic pain-consensus statement and guidelines from the Canadian Pain Society. *Pain Res Manag*; 12: 13–21. ISSN: 1203-6765.

[53] Novak V, Freimer ML, Kissel JT, et al., (2001). Autonomic impairment in painful neuropathy, *Neurology*;56:861–8. ISSN: 0028-3878

[54] Oerlemans HM, Oostendorp RA, de Boo T, van der Laan L, Severens JL, Goris JA. (2000). Adjuvant physical therapy versus occupational therapy in patients with reflex sympathetic dystrophy/ complex regional pain syndrome type I. *Arch Phys Med Rehabil*; 81: 49–56. ISSN

[55] Potter J, Higginson IJ, Scadding JW, Quigley CW. (2003). Identifying neuropathic pain in patients with head and neck cancer: use of the Leeds Assessment of Neuropathic Symptoms and Signs Scale, *J R Soc Med.*;96:379–83. ISSN: 0141-0768.

[56] Portenoy R.,(2006). Development and testing of a neuropathic pain screening questionnaire: ID Pain. *Curr Med Res Opin*;22:1555–65. ISSN: 0300-7995.

[57] Pickering G, Capriz F. (2008). Neuropathic pain in the elderly. *Psychol NeuroPsychiatr Vieil.* 6 (2) : 107-14. ISSN: 2212-4926.

[58] Pickering G. (2005). Age differences in clinical pain states. In :.*Pain in older persons.* Gibson SJ, Weiner DK, eds: IASP Press, : 67-85.8. Seattle, USA

[59] Ramachandran VS, Altschuler EL.( 2009). The use of visual feedback, in particular mirror visual feedback, in restoring brain function. *Brain*; 132: 1693–710. ISSN: 0006-8950

[60] Rolke R, Baron R, Maier C, et al.,(2006). Quantitative sensory testing in the German Research Network on Neuropathic Pain (DFNS): standardized protocol and reference values, *Pain*; 123: 231–43. ISSN: 0304-3959

[61] Scholz J, Mannion RJ, Hord DE, Griffin RS, Rawal B, et al., (2009) A novel tool for the assessment of pain: Validation in low back pain. PLoS Med 6(4):e1000047, doi:10.1371/journal.pmed.1000047;

[62] Scholz J, Broom DC, Youn DH, et al. (2005). Blocking caspase activity prevents transsynaptic neuronal apoptosis and the loss of inhibition in lamina II of the dorsal horn after peripheral nerve injury. *J Neurosci*; 25: 7317–23

[63] Sethna NF, Meier PM, Zurakowski D, Berde CB. (2007). Cutaneous sensory abnormalities in children and adolescents with complex regional pain syndromes. *Pain.*;131(1-2):153-161. ISSN: 0304-3959

[64] Serra J, Sola R, Quiles C, et al.(2009). C- nociceptors sensitized to cold in a patient with small-fiber neuropathy and cold allodynia. *Pain*; 147: 46–53. ISSN: 0304-3959

[65] Simpson DM, Brown S, Tobias J. (2008). Controlled trial of high concentration capsaicin patch for treatment of painful HIV neuropathy. *Neurology*; 70: 2305–13.ISSN: 0028-3878

[66] Siqueira SR, Alves B, Malpartida HM, Teixeira MJ, Siqueira JT. (2009). Abnormal expression of voltage-gated sodium channels Nav1.7, Nav1.3 and Nav1.8 in trigeminal neuralgia, *Neuroscience*; 164: 573–77.

[67] Steven H. Horowitz, (2007). The Diagnostic Workup of Patients with Neuropathic Pain, *Anesthesiology Clin.* 25 699–708

[68] Subedi B., Grossberg G.T. (2011). Phantom Limb Pain: Mechanisms and Treatment Approaches. *Pain Research and Treatment*,

[69] Stančák A., Kozák J, Vrba I, Tintěra J, Vrána J , Poláček H, Stančák M. (2008). Functional magnetic resonance imaging of cerebral activation during spinal cord stimulation in failed back surgery syndrome patients. *European Journal of Pain*; 12:137-48

[70] Tan EC, Zijlstra B, Essink ML, Goris RJ, Severijnen RS. (2008).Complex regional pain syndrome type I in children. *Acta Paediatr.*;97(7):875-879.

[71] Treede RD, Jensen TS, Campbell JN, Cruccu G, Dostrovsky JO, et al. (2008) Neuropathic pain: Redefinition and a grading system for clinical and research purposes. *Neurology* 70: 1630–1635. ISSN: 0028-3878

[72] Walco G.A, Dworkin R, Elliot J. Krane, LeBel, A.A. and Treede RD. (2010). Neuropathic Pain in Children: Special Considerations. *Mayo Clin Proc.*;85(3)(suppl):S33-S41. ISSN: 0025-6196

[73] Weiner DK, Rudy TE, Morrow L, Slaboda J, Lieber S. (2006).The relationship between pain, neuropsychological performance, and physical function in community-dwelling older adults with chronic low back pain. *Pain Med* ; 7 : 60-70.24. ISSN: 1526-2375

[74] Woolf CJ. In: *Hyperalgesia and Allodynia*. (1992). Willis W, ed. New York, NY: Raven Press;221-243.

[75] Woolf CJ, Bennett GJ, Doherty M, et al. (1998).Towards a mechanism-based classification of pain? *Pain*; 77: 227–29.147: 46–53. ISSN: 0304-3959

[76] Wu G, Ringkamp M, Murinson BB, et al. (2002). Degeneration of myelinated eff erent fibers induces spontaneous activity in uninjured C-fiber afferents. *J Neurosci*; 22: 7746–53. 42. ISSN: 0270-6474

[77] Ultenius C, Linderoth B, Meyerson BA, Wallin J. (2006). Spinal, NMDA receptor phosphorylation correlates with the presence of neuropathic signs following peripheral nerve injury in the rat. *Neurosci Lett*; 399: 85–90. ISSN: 0304-3940

[78] Zhuo M., Gongxiong W., Long-Jun W.( 2011). Neuronal and glial mechanisms of neuropathic pain. *Molecular Brain*,4:31. ISSN: 1756-6606

# 2

# Pharmacotherapy of Neuropathic Pain

Kishor Otari, Rajkumar Shete and Chandrashekhar Upasani
*Department of Pharmacology, Rajgad Dnyanpeeth's College of Pharmacy,*
*Bhor, Dist: Pune*
*India*

## 1. Introduction

Neuropathic pain is responsible for a significant amount of the morbidity associated with generalized and focal peripheral neuropathies (Freeman, 2005). Appropriate diagnosis and assessment are critical to the successful treatment of neuropathic pain. The diagnosis of neuropathic pain can often be challenging and diagnostic criteria are evolving. Additionally the neuropathic pain commonly coexists with other types of pain (e.g., low back pain associated with both radiculopathy and musculoskeletal abnormalities). Assessment of neuropathic pain should focus on identifying and treating the underlying disease processes and peripheral or central nervous system lesions, response to prior therapies, and comorbid conditions that can be affected by therapy. Particular attention should be paid to identifying coexisting depression, anxiety, sleep disturbances, and other adverse impacts of neuropathic pain on health-related quality of life. Both pain and its adverse effects should be reassessed frequently. Patient education and support are critical components of the successful management of neuropathic pain. Careful explanation of the cause of neuropathic pain and the treatment plan are essential. Patient's and provider's expectations regarding treatment effectiveness and tolerability must be discussed, and realistic treatment goals should be established with patients. Non-pharmacologic methods of coping with pain should be discussed, including the importance of stress reduction, good sleep hygiene, physical therapy, and other potentially useful interventions (Dworkin et al., 2007).

Although neuropathic pain occurs as a consequence of numerous peripheral and CNS disorders, a variety of agents from diverse pharmacologic classes, the so-called adjuvant analgesics, have been used to treat neuropathic pain (Table 1) (Freeman, 2005). Early recognition and aggressive management of neuropathic pain is critical to successful outcome (Hutter et al., 2007). Historically, the earliest treatment strategies for neuropathic pain were invasive in nature. It was hoped that blocking neural transmission, either temporarily using local anesthetics or permanently by surgical nerve ablation, would alleviate pain. These techniques were particularly favored in the treatment of chronic pain associated with amputations or wounds suffered by soldiers during the great wars. In 1916, Leriche suggested that vasomotor changes seen in patients with peripheral nerve damage might indicate an association between pain and abnormal vascular stimulation: this led to the use of periarterial sympathectomy in an attempt to alleviate pain. However, none of these therapies was found to be consistently successful. Oftentimes, an interdisciplinary management team provides multiple treatment modalities which includes (Chong and Bajwa, 2003):

1. Non-invasive drug therapies eg. antidepressants, antiepileptic drugs, membrane stabilizing drugs, intrathecal morphine pump systems;
2. Alternative therapies e.g. acupuncture;
3. Physical modalities eg. physical rehabilitation;
4. Psychological modalities eg. behavior modification, relaxation training;
5. Spinal cord stimulators; and
6. Invasive therapies eg. nerve blocks, ablative surgery, trigger–point injections, epidural steroids, sympathetic blocks;
7. Various surgical techniques eg. dorsal root entry zone lesions, cordotomy, and sympathectomy.

## 2. General principles

A set of principles for the use of medications will result in attenuation of symptoms in a significant majority of patients with neuropathic pain (Freeman, 2005). The majority of the randomized clinical trials (RCTs) are conducted for the certain types of patients with neuropathic pain only. Although the extent to which the results of RCTs of one type of neuropathic pain apply to other types is unknown, the extrapolation of efficacy of medications that have demonstrated efficacy in one or more types of neuropathic pain to other types of neuropathic pain is reasonable and often clinically necessary. Medications that have demonstrated efficacy in several different neuropathic pain conditions may have the greatest probability of being efficacious in additional, as yet unstudied, conditions. However, it is possible that some types of neuropathic pain respond differently to treatment. The few RCTs conducted for head-to-head comparisons of different medications that make it difficult to compare the relative efficacy and safety of many medications in neuropathic pain with different severities and duration of the treatment (Dworkin et al., 2007).

Unfortunately, there is insufficient evidence to rank medications for neuropathic pain by their degree of efficacy or safety. Given these limitations, clinicians must consider several other factors when selecting a specific medication for a patient with neuropathic pain, including (Dworkin et al., 2007):

1. The potential for adverse outcomes associated with medication-related side effects;
2. Potential drug interactions;
3. Co-morbidities that may also be relieved by the non-analgesic effects of the medication (e.g., sleep disturbance, depression, anxiety);
4. Costs associated with therapy;
5. The potential risks of medication abuse; and
6. The risks of intentional and unintentional overdose.

These potentially competing factors must be prioritized according to the specific needs of each patient with neuropathic pain. Individual variation in the response to the medications used to treat neuropathic pain is substantial and unpredictable. Although evidence-based recommendations encourage the use of specific medications, the overall approach should be recognized as a stepwise process intended to identify the medication, or medication combination, that provides the greatest pain relief and fewest side effects for a given patient. If a trial of one medication fails to adequately relieve pain or causes intolerable side effects, treatment should be discontinued and a different medication should be selected. If a medication is well tolerated and provides partial pain relief, it should be continued and a second medication with a distinct mechanism of action could be added (Dworkin et al., 2007).

In addition to potential additive analgesic benefits, combination therapy may provide analgesia more quickly by combining a medication with a rapid onset of effect with one that requires several weeks of treatment before maximum benefit is achieved. These potential advantages of combination therapy must be weighed against the possibility of additive adverse effects, drug interactions, increased cost, and reduced adherence to a more complex treatment regimen. In one of the RCTs of combination therapy in neuropathic pain, gabapentin and morphine combination provided superior pain relief to either medication alone and to placebo. However, a recent RCT evaluating nortriptyline, morphine, and their combination in patients with chronic lumbar root pain found no greater efficacy with the combination than with either medication alone or placebo (Dworkin et al., 2007).

The pharmacologic regimen for each patient should be individualized. Pharmacotherapy should be initiated with a low dose of medication, particularly in the elderly and patients susceptible to medication side effects. Most agents should be slowly titrated to minimize side effects. Since the pain of peripheral neuropathy is characteristically worse at night, it may be helpful to weight the dosing of short-acting medications to the evening hours. The onset of the therapeutic effect may be gradual and sufficient time should elapse before a conclusion is drawn, as to the success or failure of a drug. The combination of one or more drugs from a different class may result in an additive or even synergistic effect. Once patients are pain free for several months, a gradual medication taper should be considered (Freeman, 2005).

## 3. Pharmacological treatment of neuropathic pain

Pharmacotherapy of neuropathic pain is still difficult despite of new treatments, and there is no single treatment that works for all conditions and their underlying mechanisms. Given the increasing evidence for effective treatments of neuropathic pain, it is important for the clinician to know which drugs are most effective in relieving pain and associated with the fewest adverse effects and there is a need for an evidence-based algorithm to treat neuropathic pain conditions (Finnerup et al., 2005). Pharmacological management will produce the desired analgesia in some, but not all, patients. In those who fail to respond, other modalities of treatment may be considered, ranging from behavior modification and fostering of coping skills to the more major invasive medical techniques (McCleane, 2003). It is accepted that nociceptive pain may be relieved by morphine and non-steroidal anti-inflammatory drugs (NSAIDs). However, with neuropathic pain, some studies suggest analgesia with morphine (Kupers et al., 1991; Rowbotham et al., 1991) or NSAIDs (Cohen and Harris, 1987; Benedittis et al., 1992), while others demonstrate no analgesia with morphine (Arner and Meyerson1988; Eide et al., 1994) or NSAIDs (Weber et al., 1993; Max et al., 1988). However, the most neuropathic pain responds poorly to NSAIDS and opioid analgesics (Talati et al., 2011).

The mainstays of treatment of neuropathic pain are predominantly the tricyclic antidepressants (TCA's), the anticonvulsants, and the systemic local anesthetics (Talati et al., 2011; Vranken et al., 2001). Other pharmacological agents that have proven efficacious include the corticosteroids, topical therapy with substance P depletors, autonomic drugs, and N-methyl D-aspartate (NMDA) receptor antagonists (Talati et al., 2011). While many other agents may be used in treating neuropathic pain, although their use is not verified by appropriate studies. It is hoped that the rational use of drugs increases the chance of achieving analgesia in the patient with neuropathic pain. However, no one therapeutic intervention is guaranteed the success. Consequently, it may often be necessary to work ones way through a list of treatment options before analgesia is achieved. Inevitably, any relief produced may be tempered by the associated side effects of that drug so that improvement in quality of life (pain reduction, mood elevation, increased mobility, better sleep with minimal side effects from treatment) is the therapeutic goal. Poly pharmacy is a real danger, with patients staying on medication in hope of relief when none is actually apparent. Trials of medication for a defined period with assessment before and after may be more appropriate (McCleane, 2003).

Ideally, the drug choices in an evidence-based algorithm would be based on direct comparisons of one drug with another, for both efficacy and side effects. There are very few such direct comparisons available. An alternative approach is to estimate relative treatment efficacy and safety using RCT data, which is based on the number needed to treat (NNT) and number needed to harm (NNH). NNT is defined as the number of patients needed to treat with a certain drug to obtain one patient with a defined degree of pain relief, at least 50% pain relief. If 50% pain relief could not be obtained, then the number of patients reporting at least good pain relief or reporting improvement was used to calculate NNT. NNT was only calculated when the relative risk was statistically significant. NNH indicates the number of patients that need to be treated for one patient to drop out due to adverse effects. TCA's and the anticonvulsants gabapentin and pregabalin were the most frequently studied drug classes. In peripheral neuropathic pain, the lowest NNT was for TCA's, followed by opioids and the anticonvulsants gabapentin and pregabalin. Whereas, for central neuropathic pain there is limited data. NNT and NNH are currently the best way to assess relative efficacy and safety, but the need of dichotomous data estimated retrospectively for old trials, and the methodological complexity of pooling data from small cross-over and large parallel group trials, remain as limitations of NNT and NNH (Finnerup et al., 2005).

### 3.1 Drug classification (Offenbaecher and Ackenheil, 2005; Freeman, 2005; NICE clinical guideline, 2010)

| Drug class: subclass | Drugs |
|---|---|
| Opioid analgesics | Buprenorphine, co-codamol, codeine phosphate, co-dydramol, dihydrocodeine, fentanyl, morphine, oxycodone, tramadol |
| Antidepressants: | |
| Tricyclic antidepressants (TCAs) | Amitriptyline, clomipramine, desipramine, dosulepin (dothiepin), doxepin, imipramine, lofepramine, nortriptyline, trimipramine |
| Selective serotonin reuptake inhibitors (SSRIs) | Citalopram, fluoxetine, paroxetine, sertraline |
| Serotonin–norepinephrine reuptake inhibitors (SNRIs) | Duloxetine, venlafaxine |
| Anti-epileptics (anticonvulsants) | Carbamazepine, gabapentin, lamotrigine, oxcarbazepine, phenytoin, pregabalin, sodium valproate, topiramate |
| CCK antagonists | Proglumide |
| NMDA antagonists | Ketamine, dextromethorphan, riluzole, memantine, MK801 |
| Topical treatments/ membrane stabilisers | Capsaicin, lidocaine, tocainide, mexiletine |
| Miscellaneous drugs | Clonidine, cannabinoids, tetrahydrocannabinol |

Table 1. Drugs used for the treatment of neuropathic pain

### 3.1.1 Opioid analgesics

Tramadol ((1RS,2RS)-2-[(dimethylamino)methyl]-1-(3-methoxyphenyl)-cyclo-hexanol) is a synthetic opioid from the aminocyclohexanol group. It is an analgesic with opioid agonist properties that acts on the neurotransmission of noradrenaline and serotonin. In comparison with typical opioid agonists such as morphine, pethidine and the partial agonist buprenorphine, and tramadol, it rarely causes respiratory depression or physical dependence. Tramadol activates the spinal pain inhibitory system. In patients with postoperative pain of moderate or severe intensity, tramadol administered *iv* or *im* is equivalent to the analgesic potency of pethidine and pentazocine (oral route). In patients with postoperative pain of moderate intensity, tramadol analgesia (when administered *iv* in doses of 50–150 mg) is equivalent to the analgesic efficacy of morphine in doses of 5–15 mg, although during epidural administration, tramadol possesses 1/30 of the analgesic efficacy of morphine. Tramadol's main adverse reactions are nausea, dizziness, sedation, dry mouth, and sweating. Tramadol may be particularly useful for patients, who are more sensitive to the adverse effects of strong opioids (e.g., sedation, fatigue, constipation) (Leppert, 2009).

Morphine and other analogues are of limited value in most of the neuropathic pain states. Only in diabetic peripheral neuropathy oxycodone has a positive effect on pain. A special role has tramadol, which already has been proposed as an antidepressant. This unique agent combines opiate receptor agonist activity with NA reuptake inhibition, and recent research has suggested that it also has agonist activity at the 5-HT receptor. Due to this dual action it seems to have some value in the treatment of chronic neuropathic pain and can be recommended for treatment attempts (Offenbaecher and Ackenheil, 2005).

Alfentanil (active placebo), μ-opioid receptor agonist, in neuropathic pain syndromes showed significant and marked reductions of hyperalgesia to cold and also significantly reduced ongoing pain and mechanical hyperalgesia. However, no firm conclusion can be made on the long-term effect and the clinical usefullness of alfentanil (Ko et al., 2009; Offenbaecher and Ackenheil, 2005).

### 3.1.2 Antidepressants

Antidepressants and anticonvulsants are used as first-line therapy for the treatment of neuropathic pain. A meta-analysis of antidepressant use in randomized placebo-controlled trials revealed that TCAs provided at least a 50% reduction in pain intensity in 30% of individuals with neuropathic pain. Moreover, amitriptyline's a tertiary amine, is the best-studied TCA. It has been shown, in numerous randomized, blinded, placebo-controlled clinical trials, to significantly improve neuropathic pain. Amitriptyline's side effects include drowsiness, constipation, dry mouth, weight gain, and orthostatic hypotension. The secondary amines, nortriptyline and desipramine, have less troublesome side-effect profiles. The use of these agents is preferable, particularly in the elderly and side-effect prone patients, although their efficacy may not be as great. Due to possible cardiotoxicity, TCAs should be used with caution in patients with known or suspected cardiac disease (Freeman, 2005).

Current data suggest that SSRIs are not as effective as TCAs in the management of neuropathic pain. Small studies with the selective serotonin reuptake inhibitors (SSRIs), citalopram and paroxetine, have shown some improvement in symptoms of neuropathic pain in patients with painful peripheral neuropathy. The non-TCA bupropion, an Serotonin–norepinephrine reuptake inhibitor (SNRI), and a weak inhibitor of dopamine reuptake, was effective in a small, placebo-controlled trial of patients with neuropathic pain of diverse etiology, during which it was administered at 150–300 mg/day in its sustained-release form (Freeman, 2005).

The SNRIs, venlafaxine, duloxetine, and milnacipran, may prove useful in the treatment of painful diabetic peripheral neuropathy. These agents inhibit reuptake of serotonin and norepinephrine without the muscarinic, histaminic, and adrenergic side effects that accompany the use of TCAs. Venlafaxine has shown effectiveness in the treatment of neuropathic pain. In a three-way crossover trial of patients with painful neuropathy, venlafaxine 225 mg/day and imipramine 150 mg/day reduced pain scores significantly more than placebo. Surprisingly, there was no difference in the effectiveness or the side-effect profile of these two active drugs. Side effects of venlafaxine include nausea, dizziness, dry mouth, sexual dysfunction, hypertension, and irritability. Similar results were obtained with doses between 150–225 mg/day in patients with painful diabetic peripheral neuropathy (Freeman, 2005).

The SNRI duloxetine, a secondary amine, may be a more potent reuptake inhibitor in vitro than the tertiary amine SNRIs venlafaxine and milnacipran. The clinical significance of this in vitro difference in potency is uncertain. Based on evidence that duloxetine ameliorates the painful physical symptoms of depression, clinical trials were performed in patients with diabetic peripheral neuropathy. There is supporting preclinical evidence of effectiveness of duloxetine in a rodent model of neuropathic pain as well as duloxetine reverses mechanical allodynia behavior in the L5/L6 spinal nerve ligation model. Food and Drug Administration approved duloxetine for the treatment of neuropathic pain in diabetes. Common side effects of duloxetine include nausea, headache, insomnia, constipation, dry mouth, dizziness, and fatigue (Freeman, 2005).

### 3.1.3 Anti-epileptics (anticonvulsants)

Anticonvulsant agents have been used in pain management over the last few decades due to the clinical impression that they are effective in alleviating certain forms of pain for example neuropathic pain especially lancinating and burning pain (Todorovic et al., 2003), cancer pain (Keskinbora et al., 2007). Gabapentin has attracted recent attention because of its effectiveness against neuropathic pain in both controlled clinical trials and animal models (Kayser and Christensen, 2000).

It has been reported that, in addition to the anti epileptic activity, gabapentin also displays antinociceptive (Cheng and Chiou, 2006; Taylor et al., 1998), antihyperalgesic (Garry et al., 2005; Reyes-Garcia et al., 2004), and antiallodynic (Garry et al., 2005; Suzuki et al., 2005) activity in various animal pain models e.g. models of sciatic nerve chronic constriction injury (Joshi et al., 2006), spinal nerve ligation (Abdi et al., 1998; Joshi et al., 2006), diabetic neuropathy (Cheng and Chiou, 2006), acute herpes zoster infection (Cheng and Chiou, 2006), thermal injury (Garry et al., 2005; Hanesch et al., 2003) and postoperative pain (Cheng and Chiou, 2006; Field et al., 1997; Otari et al., 2010). In addition, gabapentin was shown to reduce hyperalgesia and inhibit C-fibre responses to noxious stimuli in animal models of inflammatory pain (injection of formalin or carrageenan)(Hanesch et al., 2003).

The possible mechanisms involved in the multiple therapeutic actions of gabapentin have been actively studied. Several hypothesis were raised. Despite its structural similarity to GABA, gabapentin has no discernible action at $GABA_A$ or $GABA_B$ receptors nor does it have any effect on either the uptake or degradation of GABA. However, it interacts specifically with the $\alpha_2\delta$ subunit of voltage sensitive calcium channels, a subunit ubiquitous to all calcium channel types, suggesting that the $\alpha_2\delta$ subunit is involved in the antinociceptive action of gabapentin

(Cheng and Chiou, 2006; Hanesch et al, 2003). Of the different subtypes, N-type calcium channels acquire greater functional roles after nerve injury and evidence exists for an upregulation of the $\alpha_2\delta$ -1 subunit and the N-type pore-forming $\alpha_1$ or $\beta$ subunit in this pain state (Suzuki et al., 2005). Pregabalin, a gabapentin analogue, is also effective in the management of neuropathic pain and exerts its pharmacological effects via the same mechanism as that gabapentin. The N-type calcium channel is Cav2.2 and it is unique to sensory nerve terminals in the dorsal horns of the spinal cord controlling neurotransmitter release (Cheng and Chiou, 2006). By binding to the $\alpha_2\delta$ subunit, gabapentin might affect $Ca^{2+}$ currents to modulate neurotransmitter release or neuronal excitatibility and synaptic transmission. Gabapentin reduced excitatory amino acid (glutamate and aspartate) release in the spinal cord in several pain models (Cheng and Chiou, 2006).

### 3.1.4 CCK antagonists

After systemic injection, mechanical allodynia was reduced by higher doses of cholecystokinin-B (CCK B) receptor antagonist, CI-988 (10 and 20 mg/kg). Intrathecal CI-988 (100, 200 and 500 microg) dose-dependently increased the paw withdrawal threshold in both paws after spinal cord hemisection in rats. It was suggest that up-regulation of spinal CCK may contribute to maintenance of mechanical allodynia following spinal cord injury (SCI) and that clinical application of CI-988 or similar drugs may be useful therapeutic agents for management of central neuropathic pain (Kim et al., 2009).

It was demonstrates that, the antinociception by RB 101, a complete inhibitor of enkephalin-catabolizing enzymes, was induced by elevation of extracellular levels of endogenous enkephalins, and can be extended to neuropathic pain in diabetic rats. Furthermore, blockade of CCK-B receptors potentiated antinociceptive effects elicited by RB 101. Moreover, its coadministration with CI-988, a C CK-B receptor antagonist, has been shown to strongly enhance its antinociceptive effect in normal rats (Coudore-Civiale et al., 2001).

### 3.1.5 NMDA antagonists

An NMDA antagonist, which is metabolized to dextrophan has therapeutic effects on neuropathic pain as well. In patients with posttraumatic neuropathic pain, Dextromethorphan resulted in a significant (30%) reduction of pain. Most patients (76%) experienced one of the milder to moderate dose-related adverse effects, such as light-headedness and drowsiness this may limit further use of dextromethorphan. This indicated that dextrophan is the therapeutic agent for neuropathic pain. Whereas, another NMDA receptor antagonist, memantine was also effective in patients with diabetic neuropathy and post-herpetic neuralgia (Offenbaecher and Ackenheil, 2005).

Ketamine, in patients with long lasting peripheral neuropathic pain, produced significant reduction in mean pain, measured with a visual analog scale. The clinical usefulness is however, limited by disturbing side effects mainly somnolence, light-headedness, paraesthesia etc. Ketamine in neuropathic pain syndromes showed significant and marked reductions of hyperalgesia to cold and also significantly reduced ongoing pain and mechanical hyperalgesia. However, no firm conclusion can be made on the long-term effect and the clinical usefullness of ketamine (Offenbaecher and Ackenheil, 2005).

A glycine antagonist, in patients with neuropathic pain of mixed origin, in order to reduce pain failed to show a positive effect in comparison with placebo (Offenbaecher and Ackenheil, 2005).

### 3.1.6 Miscellaneous drugs

Imidazoline receptors (IRs) are widely distributed in mammalian cells of the central (CNS) and peripheral (PNS) nervous systems, liver, kidney and heart. CR4056 is a new ligand of the imidazoline-2 sites (I2R) with efficacy in several models of pain. CR4056 is a very effective analgesic compound active in several preclinical models relevant for important human pathologies including fibromyalgia and diabetes-induced neuropathy. CR4056 has now completed preclinical development and a phase I safety study in humans has now been designed to finally develop the compound as a first I2 ligand in chronic and neuropathic pain conditions (Ferrari et al., 2011).

Administered adenosine led to a significant reduction in spontaneous pain and hyperalgesia in individuals with neuropathic pain of various etiologies. The role for intrathecal adenosine is very limited for the treatment of neuropathic pain. The cholecystokinin (CCK) 2 antagonist, L-365, in patients receiving morphine for chronic neuropathic pain was not superior (Offenbaecher and Ackenheil, 2005).

## 4. Combination pharmacotherapy

Clearly, numerous pharmacological agents are available for the treatment of neuropathic pain. The definitive drug therapy has however remained elusive. Given the limited effectiveness of current treatments, combining different drugs may result in improved results at lower doses and with fewer side effects. Many patients with neuropathic pain currently receive drug combinations, albeit in the absence of supportive evidence. Oftentimes triple drug therapy with TCA's, anti–convulsants, and a systemic local anesthetic is necessary. Occasionally, there is the patient who requires chronic opioid therapy in conjunction with the above medications. In a recent RCT, analgesia with a morphine-gabapentin combination was superior to treatment with either drug alone. In a study involving 11 patients who did not respond to gabapentin, a gabapentin-venlafaxine combination was superior to gabapentin alone. In another RCT, the addition of the neuroleptic fluphenazine to amitriptyline therapy provided no benefit. Future trials are needed to evaluate optimal drug combinations and dose ratios as well as safety, compliance, and cost-effectiveness. When patients fail failed to showresponce to systemic treatments, the implantable systems such as a spinal cord stimulator or intrathecal morphine pumps are available. Recently, the spinal cord stimulator has been shown to attenuate the augmented dorsal horn release of excitatory amino acids via a GABAergic mechanism in rats. Rarely, surgical intervention is required (Gilron et al., 2006).

## 5. Studies in progress

There are preliminary studies in neuropathic pain and fibromyalgia with very promising results. Pregabalin belongs to the class of AEDs, which modifies intracellular calcium levels and decreases norepinephrine (NE), 5-HT, and dopamine secretion. It improves diabetic neuropathy and seems to be effective in fibromyalgia patients. Another group of drugs are newer antidepressants (duloxetine and milnacipram) which inhibit NE and 5-HT reuptakte more specifically than the classic antidepressants, meaning that they have almost no effect on other transmitters and therefore have more favorable side effects. The results of these studies were reported at the 2004 Myopain Congress in Munich, Germany (Offenbaecher and Ackenheil, 2005).

Kamata and colleagues evaluated the efficacy of milnacipram, a novel serotonin-norepinephrine reuptake inhibitor, in a series of five patients with chronic pain of mixed origin. Four out of five patients experienced a pain reduction between 42% and 86% during a 12-week treatment period (Offenbaecher and Ackenheil, 2005).

In a phase II study, reported at Collegium Internationale Neuro-Psychopharmacologicum Paris in 2004, milnacipram was used in 125 patients with fibromyalgia. Administration of milnacipram either four times daily or twice daily showed that the latter was better tolerated and resulted in significant improvements of several outcome variables such as pain (37% reported a 50% reduction), fatigue, stiffness, and physical functioning. Overall, 273 adverse events were reported of which 49% were mild, 38% moderate, and 13% severe (Offenbaecher and Ackenheil, 2005).

The results of a study by Detke was presented in a congress report by Susmanon investigations on duloxetine in patients with diabetic neuropathy. Duloxetine is a potent and balanced dual reuptake inhibitor of both 5-HT and NE, possessing comparable affinities in binding to NE and 5-HT transport sites, in contrast to most other dual-reuptake inhibitors. In 457 patients with diabetic neuropathy receiving placebo or three different doses of duloxetine in a 12-weeks, multicentre, double-blind study, 60 mg and the 120 mg dose were significantly more effective in reducing 24-hour pain. In the highest dose, patients displayed more side effects, such as nausea, somnolence, dizziness, and increased appetite. This clinical results provided evidence that duloxetine 60 mg/day and duloxetine 60 mg BID is effective in the treatment of pain associated with diabetic neuropathy. These positive results of duloxetine on pain were further supported by a currently published study by Goldstein and colleagues. Data from 3 different studies investigating primarily the effect of duloxetine on mood in patients with major depression were analysed concerning painful symptoms, as secondary outcome in these studies. The authors found that compared to placebo, duloxetine reduces significantly painful physical symptoms in these patients (Offenbaecher and Ackenheil, 2005).

Crofford and colleagues investigated the efficacy and safety of pregabalin in 529 patients with fibromyalgia. In this multicenter study three different doses of pregabalin 150 mg, 300 mg, and 450 mg were compared with placebo over an 8-week period. It was found that, the highest pregabalin dose produced a significant pain reduction (change from baseline of two points on a visual analog scale). Additionally, other outcome (eg, sleep quality, fatigue, and health-related QOL) improved as well. However, a high proportion of the patients reported side effects such as dizziness, somnolence, headaches, and others (Offenbaecher and Ackenheil, 2005).

## 6. Conclusion

In clinical practice the most frequently prescribed drugs in chronic neuropathic pain are classic TCAs and AEDs, both of them have the well-known side effects, which limit their long-term administration (Offenbaecher and Ackenheil, 2005).

However new studies using randomized, double-blind, placebo controlled trials are increasing to support evidence based algorithm to treat neuropathic pain conditions. The neuropathic pain is a devastating chronic condition that generally can be diagnosed by history and findings on physical examination. For some neuropathic pain syndromes, available treatments are tolerable and afford meaningful relief to a considerable proportion of patients. Nevertheless, many patients report intractable and severe pain and better treatment strategies are desperately needed. Furthermore, the coexistence of neuropathic, nociceptive, and occasionally, idiopathic pain in the same patient leads pharmacotherapy difficult. Also, neuropathic pain has historically been classified according to its etiology (e.g.

painful diabetic neuropathy, trigeminal neuralgia, spinal cord injury) without regard for the presumed mechanism(s) underlying the specific symptoms. Hence, currently, no consensus on the optimal management of neuropathic pain exists and practices vary greatly worldwide. The treatment of neuropathic pain is largely empirical, often relying heavily on data from small, generally poorly-designed clinical trials or anecdotal evidence.

It is still reassuring, however, to realise that in the future we have the prospect of additional agents with more specific sodium channel blocking effects, calcium channel blockers and new generation anticonvulsants and capitalise on the major expansion in knowledge generated from the work of the basic scientists. The field of neuropathic pain research and treatment is in the early stages of development, with many goals yet to be achieved. In particular, future laboratory, clinical, and epidemiologic research into pathogenesis, treatment, and prevention of neuropathic pain is expected as well as improved dissemination of new information to health professionals and the public. Over the years to come, many upcoming advances are expected in the basic and clinical science of neuropathic pain as well as in the implementation of improved therapies for patients who continue to experience these devastating conditions.

Recently, the problem has been recognized—there is possible shift from rheumatology to psychiatry—and newer studies have been published or are still in progress. These newer drugs—on the one hand, specific dual NE/5-HT reuptake inhibitors, and on the other hand newer AEDs—are promising in terms of efficacy and fewer side effects (Offenbaecher and Ackenheil, 2005).

## 7. References


Abdi, S.; Lee, D.H. & Chung, J M. (1998). The anti-allodynic effects of amitriptyline, gabapentin, and lidocaine in a rat model of neuropathic pain. *Anesthesia & Analgesia*, 87, 1360–1366.

Arner, S. & Meyerson, BA. (1988). Lack of analgesic effect of opioids on neuropathic and idiopathic forms of pain. *Pain*, 33, 11 - 23.

Benedittis G.D.; Besana F. & Lorenzetti A. (1992). A new topical treatment for acute herpetic neuralgia and post-herpetic neuralgia: the aspirin / diethyl ether mixture. An open label study plus a double-blind controlled clinical trial. *Pain*, 48, 383 - 390.

Cheng, J.K. & Chiou, L.C. (2006). Mechanisms of the antinociceptive action of gabapentin. *Journal of Pharmacological Sciences*, 100, 471–486.

Chong, M.S. & Bajwa, Z.H. (2003). Diagnosis and Treatment of Neuropathic Pain. *Journal of Pain and Symptom Management*, 25 (5S), S4-S11.

Cohen, K.L. & Harris, S. (1987). Efficacy and safety of non-steroidal anti-inflammatory drugs in the therapy of diabetic neuropathy. *Archives of internal medicine* , 147, 1442 -1444.

Coudore-Civiale, M.A.; Meen, M.; Fournie-Zaluski, M.C.; Boucher, M.; Roques, B.P. & Eschalier A. (2001). Enhancement of the effects of a complete inhibitor of enkephalin-catabolizing enzymes, RB 101, by a cholecystokinin-B receptor antagonist in diabetic rats. British Journal of Pharmacology, 133(1),179-185.

Eide, P.K.; Jorum, E. & Stubhaug, A. (1994). Relief of post herpetic neuralgia with the N-methyl-D-aspartate receptor antagonist ketamine: a double-blind, cross-over comparison with morphine and placebo. *Pain*, 58, 347 - 354.

Ferrari, F.; Fiorentino, S.; Mennuni, L.; Garofalo, P.; Letari, O.; Mandelli, S.; Giordani, A.; Lanza, M. & Caselli, G. (2011). Analgesic efficacy of CR4056, a novel imidazoline-2 receptor ligand, in rat models of inflammatory and neuropathic pain. *Journal of Pain Research*, 4, 111–125.

Field, M.J.; Holloman, E.F.; McCleary, S., Hughes, J. & Singh, L. (1997). Evaluation of gabapentin and *S*- (1)-3-isobutylgaba in a rat model of postoperative pain. *The Journal of Pharmacology and Experimental Therapeutics*, 282 (3), 1242–1246.

Finnerup, N.B.; Otto, M.; McQuay, H.J.; Jensen, T.S. & Sindrup, S.H. (2005). Algorithm for neuropathic pain treatment: An evidence based proposal. *Pain*, 118, 289–305.

Freeman, R. (2005). The Treatment of Neuropathic Pain. *CNS Spectrums*, 10 (9), 698-706.

Garry, E.M.; Delaney, A.; Andersona, H.A.; Sirinathsinghji E.C.; Clapp R.H.; Martin W.J.; Kinchington, P.R.; Krah, D.L..; Abbadie, C. & Fleetwood-Walker, S.M. (2005). Varicella zoster virus induces neuropathic changes in rat dorsal root ganglia and behavioral reflex sensitisation that is attenuated by gabapentin or sodium channel blocking drugs. *Pain*, 118, 97–111.

Gilron, I.; Watson, C.P.N.; Cahill, C.M. & Moulin, D.E. (2006). Neuropathic pain: a practical guide for the clinician. *Canadian Medical Association Journal*, 175(3), 265-275.

Hanesch, U.; Pawlak, M. & McDougall, J.J. (2003). Gabapentin reduces the mechanosensitivity of fine afferent nerve fibers in normal and inflamed rat knee joints. *Pain*, 104, 363–366.

Hutter, J.; Reich-Weinberger, S.; Hitzl, W. & Stein, H.J. (2007). Sequels 10 years after thoracoscopic procedures for benign disease. *European Journal of Cardio-Thoracic Surgery*, 32(3), 409-411.

Joshi, S.K.; Hernandez, G.; Mikusa, J.P.; Zhu, C.Z.; Zhong, C.; Salyers, A.; Wismer, C.T.; Chandran, P.; Decker, M.W. & Honore, P. (2006). Comparison of antinociceptive actions of standard analgesics in attenuating capsaicin and nerve-Injury induced mechanical hypersensitivity. *Neuroscience*, 143, 587–596.

Kayser, V. & Christensen, D. (2000). Antinociceptive effect of systemic gabapentin in mononeuropathic rats depends on stimulus characteristics and level of test integration. *Pain*, 88, 53–60.

Keskinbora, K.; Pekel, A.F. & Isik, A. (2007). Gabapentin and an opioid combination versus opioid alone for the management of neuropathic cancer pain: A randomized open trial. *Journal of Pain and Symptom Management*, 34(2), 183–189.

Kim, J.; Kim, J.H.; Kim, Y.; Cho, H.Y.; Hong, S.K. & Yoon, Y.W. (2009). Role of spinal cholecystokinin in neuropathic pain after spinal cord hemisection in rats. Neuroscience Letter, 462(3), 303-307.

Ko, M.C.; Woods, J.H.; Fantegrossi, W.E.; Galuska, C.M.; Wichmann, J. & Prinssen, E.P. 2009. Behavioral Effects of a Synthetic Agonist Selective for Nociceptin/ Orphanin FQ Peptide Receptors in Monkeys. *Neuropsychopharmacology*, 34, 2088–2096.

Kupers, R.C.; Konings, H.; Adriaensen, H. & Gybels, J.M. (1991). Morphine differentially affects sensory and affective pain ratings in neurogenic and idiopathic forms of pain. *Pain* , 47, 5 - 12.

Leppert, W. (2009). Tramadol as an analgesic for mild to moderate cancer pain. *Pharmacological reports*, 61, 978-992.

Macres, S.M. (2003). Understanding Neuropathic Pain. *Pain Medicine*, 33 (1), 1-8.

Max, M.B.; Schafer, S.C.; Culnane, M.S.; Dubner, R. & Gracely, R.H. (1988). Association of pain relief with drug side effects in post herpetic neuralgia: a single-dose study of clonidine, codeine, ibuprofen and placebo. *Clinical pharmacology and therapeutics*, 43, 363 - 371.

McCleane, G. (2003). Pharmacological management of neuropathic pain. *CNS Drugs*, 17(14), 1031-1043.

McQuay, H.; Carroll, D.; Jadad, A.R.; Wiffen, P. & Moore, A. (1995). Anticonvulsant drugs for management of pain: a systematic review. *British Medical Journal*. 21, 311(7012), 1047-1052.

NICE clinical guideline 96. (2010). Neuropathic pain: the pharmacological management of neuropathic pain in adults in non-specialist settings. www.nice.org.uk/guidance/CG96.

Offenbaecher, M. &Ackenheil, M. (2005). Current Trends in Neuropathic Pain Treatments with Special Reference to Fibromyalgia. *CNS Spectrums*, 10 (4), 285-297.

Otari, K.V.; Taranalli, A.D.; Shete, R.V.; Singh, V.P. & Harpallani, A.N. (2010). Evaluation of modulatory role of gabapentin in incisional pain and inflammation. *Pharmacologyonline*, 2, 524-532.

Reyes-Garcia, G.; Caram-Salas, N.L.; Medina-Santillan, R. & Granados-Soto, V. (2004). Oral administration of B vitamins increases the antiallodynic effect of gabapentin in the Rat. *Proceedings of the Western Pharmacology Society*, 47, 76–79.

Rowbotham, M.C.; Reisner-Keller, L.A. & Fields, H.L. (1991). Both intravenous lidocaine and morphine reduce the pain of post herpetic neuralgia. *Neurology*, 41, 1024 - 1028.

Suzuki, R.; Rahman, W.; Rygh, L.J.; Webber, M.; Hunt, S.P. & Dickenson, A.H. (2005). Spinal-supraspinal serotonergic circuits regulating neuropathic pain and its treatment with gabapentin. *Pain*, 117, 292–303.

Talati, G.; Shah, S.; Trivedi, V. & Chorawala, M. (2011). Neuropathic pain: molecular mechanisms and treatment. *Research Journal of Pharmaceutical Science and Biotechnology*, 1(2), 27-34.

Taylor, C.P.; Gee, N.S.; Su, T.Z.; Kocsis, J.D.; Welty, D.F.; Brown, J.P.; Dooley, D.J.; Boden, P. & Singh, L. (1998). A summary of mechanistic hypotheses of gabapentin pharmacology. *Epilepsy Research*, 29 (3), 231–246.

Todorovic, S.M.; Rastogi, A.J. & Todorovic, V.J. (2003). Potent analgesic effects of anticonvulsants on peripheral thermal nociception in rats. *British Journal of Pharmacology*, 140, 255–260.

Vranken, J.H.; van der Vegt, M.H.; Zuurmond, WW, Pijl, A.J. & Dzoljic, M. (2001). Continuous brachial plexus block at the cervical level using a posterior approach in the management of neuropathic cancer pain. *Regional Anesthesia and Pain Medicine* , 26(6), 572-575.

Weber, H.; Holme, I. &Amlie, E. (1993). The natural course of acute sciatica with nerve root symptoms in a double-blind placebo-controlled trial evaluating the effect of piroxicam. *Spine*, 11, 1433 - 1438.

3

# Intravenous Therapies in the Management of Neuropathic Pain: A Review on the Use of Ketamine and Lidocaine in Chronic Pain Management

Harsha Shanthanna
*McMaster University, Michael DeGroote School of Medicine*
*Canada*

## 1. Introduction

Neuropathic Pain is a term referred to "pain arising as a direct consequence of a lesion affecting the somatosensory system". As a first line option, oral medications are mostly used, as they are easily available, relatively safe, and do not need much resources. They include antidepressants in the form of tricyclics, newer selective reuptake inhibitors of serotonin and norepinephrine, gabapentin, pregabalin etc. Although neuropathic pain conditions do share some common clinical features, they are quite diverse when considered individually according to their etiology and pathogenesis. Hence not all patients and not all types of neuropathic pain respond to such oral therapy. In practice patients are given a form of such neuropathic pain medication along with or without an opioid, depending upon the extent of pain that the patient suffers. Opioids are potent analgesics but are not a good choice for neuropathic pain conditions. With time the clinician is left with fewer alternatives and furthermore, with the the increasing knowledge that escalation of opioid therapy will perhaps lead to hyperalgesia and tolerance, it becomes necessary to explore other options. Among the other options one can always consider to explore treatment with intravenous medication such as Ketamine, Lidocaine, and Magnesium etc. This chapter would highlight the use of ketamine and lidocaine in the form of drug profile, the pharmacological basis behind its use, strategies to use, important side effects and limitations and available evidence base, including a review of randomised controlled studies. Both are considered separately in two different parts. References for both the parts are given at the end, in separate sections.

## Part A: Ketamine

**1. Ketamine** is a potent anesthetic and analgesic compound with unique actions. It is a phencyclidine (PCP), anesthetic compound with its chemical name being 2-O-chlorophenyl-2-methylamino- cyclohexanone. It contains an asymmetric carbon atom and exists as 2 isomers {(R) and (S)}, of which the (S) isomer is the more potent general anesthetic and NMDA antagonist. Commercially available ketamine formulations are a racemic mixture of S (+) and R (-) preserved in benzethonium chloride (Orser, 1997; Ben Ari, 2007). Animal studies has shown that the affinity at the phencyclidine binding site of S (+) ketamine at the NMDA receptor is four fold that of R(-). Studies in rats and mice have demonstrated that the S (+) form is five times more hypnotic and three times more analgesic than the R (-) raceme (White, 1985). The incidence of side effects is although similar, overall it is theoretically less, as you need less S ketamine for a therapeutic action and the side effects are observed to be proportional to their blood levels.

Ketamine is unique because no other drug combines the property of anesthetic, analgesic and amnesic properties. The search for a PCP compound with less hallucinogenic side effects led to ketamine (CI-581), first synthezised in 1962 by Calvin Stevens at Parke-Davis and Co, and introduced into clinical practice during 1970 after investigation from Corssen and Domino in 1964 on human volunteers (Sinner & Graf, Sabia, 2011). Apart from the property of dissociative anesthesia, its analgesic effects have been widely investigated, in both experimental and human studies. The analgesic properties of ketamine primarily exist because of its property to block NMDA receptor in a non-competitive fashion. Other clinically known NMDA-receptor blockers include dextromethorphan, dextrorphan, memantine, and amantadine. There are other mechanisms of analgesia which could be partly responsible for the actions of ketamine. Ketamine is also active at opioid, norepinephrine, serotonin, and muscarinic cholinergic receptors; it acts by inhibiting serotonin and dopamine reuptake and inhibits voltage-gated Na+ and K+ channels (Okon, 2007). Indeed, some studies suggest that analgesic effects of Ketamine are actually due to its activation of monoaminergic descending inhibitory pathways, rather than NMDA receptor (Okon, 2007). To understand its mechanism one has to also understand the role of NMDA receptors, at least briefly, as related to pain mechanisms.

## 2. NMDA receptor, central sensitization and chronic pain

1. NMDA receptors are known to be involved in the development of wind up phenomenon and generation of central sensitization and hence chronic pain.
2. There is increasing evidence that NMDA receptors are also involved in peripheral sensitization and visceral pain.
3. Evidence shows that Ketamine primarily acts at NMDA receptors but also has actions at other sites.

### 2.1 Pain is mediated through C (unmyelinated) and A-delta (thinly myelinated) fibres

The primary excitatory neurotransmitter released via C fibres is Glutamate. This is the major excitatory neurotransmitter in the mammalian nervous system and modulates several functions through subtypes of glutaminergic receptor: the *N*-methyl-D-aspartate (NMDA) subtype, the kainite, the AMPA (l-amino-3-hydroxy-5-methylsoxasole-propionic acid) subtype, and the metabotropic subtype (Bennett, 2000). NMDA receptor is also called "coincidence detector", as several events must combine to activate it. Apart from glutamate, glycine is also needed as a co-agonist (Carpenter, 1999). NMDARs display a number of unique properties that distinguish them from other ligand-gated ion channels. First, the receptor controls a cation channel that is highly permeable to monovalent ions and calcium. Second, simultaneous binding of glutamate and glycine, the co-agonist, is required for efficient activation of NMDAR. Third, at resting membrane potential the NMDAR channels are blocked by extracellular magnesium and open only on simultaneous depolarization and agonist binding, thus both depolarization of the postsynaptic neuron and presynaptic release of glutamate and glycine are required for maximum current flow through the NMDAR channel. The response of ionotropic glutamate receptors to agonists is usually potentiated after phosphorylation.

**Wind-up** is a progressive, frequency-dependent facilitation or increase in the magnitude of C-fiber evoked responses, of the responses of a neurone observed on the application of repetitive (usually electrical) stimuli of constant intensity. **Central sensitization** refers to enhanced excitability of dorsal horn neurons and is characterized by increased spontaneous activity, decrease in response threshold, enlarged receptive field (RF) areas, and an increase in responses evoked by large and small caliber primary afferent fibers (Jun Li, 1999; Cook, 1987). Sensitization of dorsal horn neurons often occurs following tissue injury and inflammation and is believed to contribute to hyperalgesia.

### 2.2 NMDA activation

Because it is a transmembrane protein, it spans the electric field generated by the membrane potential. The magnesium binding site within the receptor is physically located within this electric field. As the cell is depolarized, the negative field effect weakens and in this phase, when the magnesium is absent, $Ca^{2+}$, $Na^{+}$ and $K^{+}$ -ions flow through the channel. Magnesium ions are rapidly substituted by next set of magnesium ions during repolarization. The $Ca^{2+}$ influx is crucial for the induction of the NMDA receptor-dependent long-term potentiation (LTP), which is thought to underlie neuronal plasticity, including development of central sensitization, learning and memory. The activation of the NMDA receptor leads to a $Ca^{2+}$ /calmodulin-mediated activation of NO synthetase, which plays a crucial role in nociception and neurotoxicity. The primary endogenous neurotransmitter active at NMDA-R is glutamate, the main EAA. It is likely that glutamate facilitates the activation of NMDAR, by causing the intracellular elevation of calcium, leading to a cascade of excitatory events. The sequence of these intracellular signaling events is complex. However, they seem to result in the activation of protein kinase C and elevation of levels of nitrous oxide, which in turn, leads to enhanced release of other EAAs (Sinner & Graf, 2008; Petrenko, 2003; Zhou, 2011).

### 2.3 Peripheral NMDA receptors and their involvement

Several studies have demonstrated the presence of peripheral NMDA receptors which are involved with pain. Local injections of glutamate or NMDA agonists result in nociceptive behaviors that can be decreased by peripheral administration of NMDAR antagonists (Zhou, 1996). Pederson found that ketamine infiltration had only brief local analgesic effects, but several measures of pain and hyperalgesia were unaffected. Therefore, a clinically relevant effect of peripheral ketamine in acute pain seems unlikely. The local anesthetic action of ketamine can also result from its blocking of cations, and it has been demonstrated that it enhances the local anesthetic and analgesic actions of bupivacaine used for infiltration anesthesia in a postoperative setting (Tverskoy, 1996) and also the development of primary and secondary hyperalgesia after an experimental burn injury (Warnke, 1997). Topical application of ketamine ointment has been recently reported to reduce pain intensity and to attenuate allodynia in patients with an acute early dystrophic stage of complex regional pain syndrome type I (Ushida, 2002).

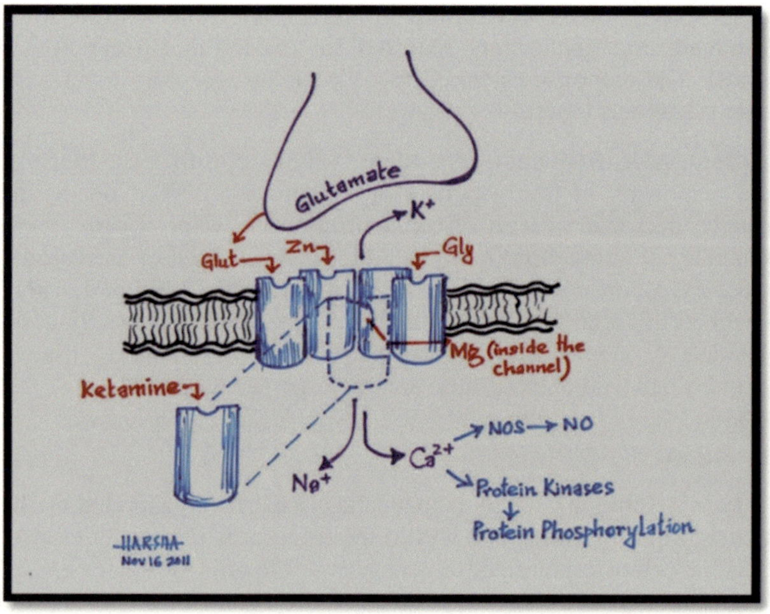


Fig. 1. NMDA Receptor and Mediators involved

## 3. Pharmacokinetics and pharmacodynamics

The bioavailability after IV administration is about 90%, whereas bioavailability after oral and rectum administrations is 16%, indicating significant first-pass effect by the liver. Particularly, oral administration of ketamine is accompanied by extensive first-pass metabolism, and the plasma levels of (R and S)-norketamine are about three times higher than the levels produced by IV or IM administration (Yanagihara 2003). Nor Ketamine, which is excreted in urine, is thought to have about 30% of the analgesic potency of the parent drug (Sinner & Graf, 2008). Ketamine is soluble in both water and lipids. Because of its high lipid solubility, it crosses the blood-brain barrier rapidly leading to the onset of action within 1-3 minutes and is rapidly redistributed (Sabia, 2011). Brain to plasma ratio for ketamine is estimated to be 6.5:1, suggesting ketamine's preferential accumulation in the brain (Orser, 1997). Timing to maximum pain relief remains a controversial issue, since it depends on the mechanism of the pain. In the Mercadante et al series (Mercandate, 2010), maximum pain relief after a single intravenous dose occurred between 30 and 60 minutes after the infusion. Elimination due to metabolism has a half-life of 2 to 3 h. The plasma clearance is 15–20 ml/kg per minute in adults and higher for S (+)-ketamine than for the enantiomer. It has a large volume of distribution in the steady state (Vss: 3.1 L/kg), owing to its low plasma-protein binding of 27%. Because of the large Vss and relatively rapid clearance, it is clinically possible to administer ketamine as an infusion at 25 to 100 µg/min (Sabia, 2011). With scheduled administration, a steady state is achieved in 12-15 hours. The initial metabolite is norketamine and is produced by the N-demethylation of ketamine, which is mediated by the hepatic cytochrome P450 enzymes (Goldberg, 2010). This is shown to be enantioselective, with the N-demethylation of (S)-ketamine proceeding faster than that of (R)-ketamine (Kharasch, 1992). A dose reduction in patients with hepatic impairment is advised due to the prolonged duration of action. In renal failure, dose increases may be considered. The urinary excretion of unmetabolized drug is approximately 4%. In forensic medicine, ketamine use can be detected in the urine for about 3 days. Concentration ranges for ketamine in urine have been reported as low as 10 ng/ml and up to 25 µg/ml.

| | |
|---|---|
| Chemical Name | 2O-chlorophenyl-2-methylamino-cyclohexanone |
| Chemical Structure | C 13 H 16 ClNO |
| Molecular Weight | 274.4 M |
| Melting Point | 258°C and 261°C |
| Solubility | Both lipid and water soluble |
| Isomers | S(+) and R(-) isomers<br>S 3-4 times more potent than R as an anesthetic |
| **BIOAVAILABILITY** | |
| Intramuscular | 93% |
| Nasal | 25%-50% |
| Oral | 17% |
| Protein Binding | 20%–30% |
| **ONSET OF EFFECTS** | |
| Intravenous | seconds |
| Intramuscular | 1-5 mins |
| Nasal | 5-10 mins |
| Oral | 15-20 mins |
| **HALF LIFE** | |
| Alpha | Alpha half-life (2–4 min) |
| Beta | Beta half-life 8–16 min (redistribution) |
| Terminal/elimination | 2.5 to 3 hrs |

Table 1. Pharmacological Properties

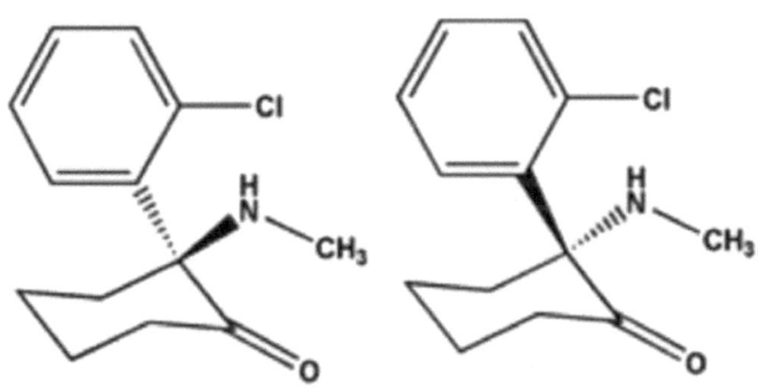


Fig. 2. Chemical Structure of Ketamine

The observation that oral administration is associated with higher serum concentrations of the main metabolite of ketamine, norketamine, compared to other routes of administration has led to the idea that norketamine contributes to the analgesic effects of ketamine (Fischer, 2010). The oral bioavailability of ketamine after a single oral dose is about one fifth of the availability after an intravenous injection. When ketamine is administered as a racemic mixture, both S-norketamine and R-norketamine is formed. Analgesic effects of ketamine were observed with plasma levels of 100–200 ng/ml (sum of S- and R-isomer) following intramuscular and intravenous administration. Effective analgesia following oral dose occurs at much lower concentrations of ketamine (40 ng/ml) (Grant et al., 1981). Clinical studies have shown that with a prolonged infusion of ketamine the ratio of ketamine to norketamine serum levels remains constant at 3:14 (Ebert, 1997). It is also not sure why some patients do not respond to ketamine and in particular to oral ketamine. Rabben and Oye found a positive correlation between a long pain history and lack of analgesic effect and also between a short pain history and a long-term analgesic effect of low-dose ketamine. This finding was also observed in the study of Mathiesen et al, where patients suffering from pain for more than 5 years did not observe any analgesic effects. These results indicate that pain mechanisms are subject to alterations with time and that these alterations involve transition from NMDA to non-NMDA receptor-mediated transmission in central pain pathways.

## 4. Mechanisms of action of ketamine

### 4.1 Ketamine blocks the NMDA channel by 2 distinct mechanisms

1) it blocks the open channel and there by reduces channel mean open time, and 2) it decreases the frequency of channel opening by an allosteric mechanism (Orser, 1997). But the precise interactions of ketamine with NMDARs are still being elucidated (Orser, 1997; Kohrs, 1998). The main interaction is supposed to result from its binding to the phencyclidine receptor in the NMDA channel and thus inhibiting the glutamate activation of the channel in a non-competitive manner (Kohrs, 1998). However the complete spectrum of effects on NMDARs is not completely clear. There may be some actions mediated differently, which are selectively active at low doses. Drugs like memantine and amantadine have no appreciable anesthetic or analgesic properties but still inhibit NMDARs. This dual mechanism may be clinically relevant in treating patients with low dose and high dose ketamine, and my may in fact act through different pathways apart from molecular mechanisms.

### 4.2 Other mechanisms of possible ketamine actions

1. Opioid: It is said to be an antagonist at mu and agonist at kappa receptors (Sinner & Graf, 2008; White, 1982).
2. Ketamine is known to produce local anesthetic effect similar to lidocaine and bupivacaine. Spinal administration of ketamine mixed with epinephrine produces motor and sensory block without respiratory depression or hypotension, even in humans, but are associated with central effects unlike in dogs. This has been used in war casualties.
3. Activation or increase in the activity of descending monoaminergic system (serotonergic).
4. Effects on muscarinic cholinergic receptors are not shown to be responsible for analgesia.

## 5. A practical algorithm for ketamine in chronic pain

For long term use

1. Monitor for Ketamine induced changes in cognition, memory and mood disturbances.
2. Monitor for Ketamine addiction, using the same guidelines as opioids.
3. Long term neuraxial use is not advised as it is supposed to be associated with side effects.

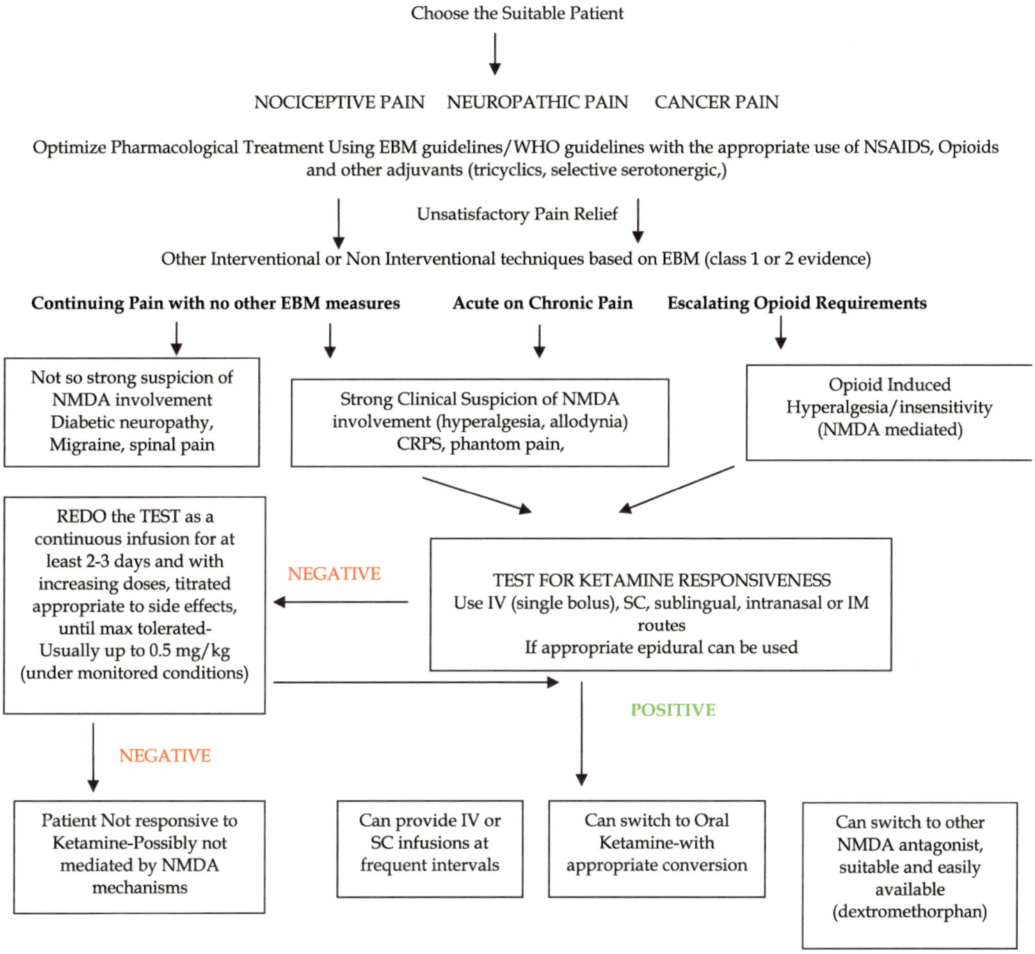


## 6. An analysis of RCT's of parenteral ketamine

The evidence for the use of Ketamine in chronic, neuropathic pain consists of RCT's, case reports, case series, retrospective studies and experimental studies. RCT's are considered as "level 2 evidence", as per the EBM standards. We performed a search of Pubmed and EMBASE to look for RCT's using ketamine for chronic pain. We also included studies on cancer pain management. Limits were put on English language and human controlled trials. Mesh terms used were as following: 'ketamine', 'administration', 'chronic pain', 'neuropathic pain', 'cancer pain', 'intravenous', 'subcutaneous', 'intramuscular'. Articles describing a study based on animal research and research about acute postoperative pain and reviews were excluded by entering the term 'NOT' in the search strategy. Only abstracts were not included. We also cross referenced our search results with previous review articles (Hocking, 2003; Bell 2009). Finally a total of 33 articles were selected. Out of them 3 articles were excluded: Eide (1997): this is an N=1 trial, Hagelberg (2010): this trial was just looking at how antibiotic levels affect ketamine levels (the identical dose of ketamine was used in both arms of the trial), Neisters (2011): experimental study on human volunteers. Most included small numbers of patients with a variety of study objectives, designs and outcome measurements. None of the included studies had a high quality methodological design. Due to the above reasons and with the heterogeneity of data, it was not possible to perform a quantitative analysis.

In total we obtained 30 studies. Categorisation according to clinical diagnosis showed; 3 studies of CRPS, 2 were on fibromyalgia, 2 on ischemic pain, 2 on post herpetic neuralgia, 3 on peripheral neuropathic pain, 1 on post traumatic pain, 3 studies on various chronic neuropathic pain conditions, 2 on post nerve injury pain, 2 on phantom limb pain, 2 on whiplash, 1 on odontolgia and TMJ pain, 3 on spinal cord injury pain, 1 on post stroke pain, 1 on migraine treatment and prophylaxis, 1 on cancer pain, 1 was an experimental study. According to route of administration there were: 1 study on subcutaneous infusion, 2 studies on intranasal use, 1 study on intramuscular use, and a total of 26 studies on intravenous use.

| Author/ Year | Design | Patient population and numbers | Design/ Methodology | Outcomes | Withdrawal/Side Effects |
|---|---|---|---|---|---|
| Carr (2004) | DB RCT PLC | N=22; Chronic pain; currently on 24hr opioid regimens | Ketamine intranasal spray (Ketamine HCL 10%) vs. placebo (NS) 1-5 sprays q90s x 5 for breakthrough pain (BTP) | Significantly lower BTP after IN Ketamine vs. placebo; pain relief up to 60 min. No patient in treatment arm required usual breakthrough pain meds vs. 7 who did in treatment arm | 4 patients reported a change in taste, 2 experienced increase in blood pressure, 1 reported nasal passage irritation and rhinorrhea |
| Huge (2010) | DB RCT | N=16; Chronic neuropathic syndromes | Ketamine 0.2mg/kg intranasal vs. Ketamine 0.4mg/kg intranasal five sprays each nostril x 1 | Significant decrease in resting pain in both groups up to 1 hr after application on 100 point pain scale; no change in quantitative sensory testing | 75% of subjects reported vertigo, 70% reported sedation; 60% reported difficulty concentrating |

Table 2. RCT's of Intranasal Route

### 6.1 Intranasal route

This route was used in 2 studies, breakthrough pain and various neuropathic pain conditions. This is also utilised in some outpatient clinics to help identify patient's responsiveness to ketamine without involving the logistics and preparation as necessary for IV ketamine infusion. Both studies were positive with respect to ketamine's analgesic actions. Huge studies the use of intranasal S ketamine randomised into 2 different doses (0.2 mg/kg and 0.4 mg/kg). Plasma concentrations of S Ketamine and S norketamine were also studied. The analgesic effects co-related with maximum plasma range of metabolites for both doses after which it decreased.

Intranasal ketamine can act similar to a parenteral route as it can bypass the hepatic metabolism. Apart from the known side effects, intranasal use can cause transient change in taste, rhinorrhea, irritation of nasal passage (Carr, 2004).

### 6.2 Intramuscular route

IM use is considered parenteral and for all reasons it is considered similar to IV ketamine administration, except that the onset of effect can be prolonged. The only study was done on TMJ pain patients suspected of myofascial pain. Ketamine injection was given as a single dose injection into the most painful part of masseter at a dose of 0.2 ml, in comparison to placebo. There were no differences in pain scores except a minor effect on jaw opening. Although the reason for injection at the local painful site is not provided, it may be assumed that a local or peripheral site of action was considered.

| Author/ Year | Design | Patient population and numbers | Design/ Methodology | Outcomes | Withdrawal/ Side Effects |
|---|---|---|---|---|---|
| Castrillon (2008) | DB RCT | N=14; Myofascial TMJ syndrome | Ketamine injection (0.2 ml) into masseter vs NS injection x1 | No difference in VAS pain questionnaire scores | None |

Table 3. RCTs of Intramuscular Route

### 6.3 Subcutaneous route

The subcutaneous route is also considered parenteral. Although there have been many case reports and case series using sc route, there was only one RCT. Nicolodi et al used sc

| Author/ Year | Design | Patient population and numbers | Design/ Methodology | Outcomes | Withdrawal/ Side Effects |
|---|---|---|---|---|---|
| Nicolodi (1995) | DB RCT PLC | N=17; Chronic migraine headaches | Ketamine (80 mcg/kg) subcut vs Placebo (NS) subcut daily x 3 weeks | Significant decrease in frequency and severity of migraine attacks | "Most" patients experienced mild side effects |

Table 4. RCTs of Subcutaneous Route

ketamine as bolus and 3 times daily for acute migraine and its prophylaxis, compared to placebo infusion. Ketamine gave marked pain relief in both acute situation and as a prophylactic. However, subcutaneous administration of ketamine is associated with significant side effects. Apart from the central side effects such as hallucinations and delirium, peripheral side effects at the injection site are common. Ketamine is an irritant and requires daily changing of injection site (Hocking, 2003). Itching and painful indurations at the injection site were also observed by Eide et al (1995). Heparin ointment is supposed to help with this troublesome side effect (Klepstad, 1997)

### 6.4 Intravenous administration of Ketamine

Out of 26 studies of IV ketamine, 1 was experimental. Oga demonstrated that pain reduction with ketamine is correlated with ketamine induced changes in hallucinatory behaviour and excitement as measured by brief psychiatric rating scale (BPRS).

#### 6.4.1 Whiplash disorder

Ketamine was found to be beneficial in both the studies. Both were done by Lemming et al. The exact nature of pathology in whiplash is still unknown. Interventional treatments such cervical facet denervation has been found to be very effective in many patients. The utility of ketamine in this group of patients needs further studies with well defined inclusion criteria.

#### 6.4.2 Pain of vascular origin

Two studies (Mitchell, 2002; Perrson, 1998) examined the effect of ketamine on critical limb ischemia and arteriosclerosis obliterans respectively. Both had positive results. The numbers treated were small (total N=16). Ketamine at a dose of 0.45 mg/kg fared better than Morphine 10 mg in arteriosclerosis patients.

#### 6.4.3 Fibromyalgia

This is perhaps the least understood of neuropathic pain conditions despite being quite prevalent. Although the etiology is unknown the pathology does involve myofascial and connective tissue layers, at least in terms of its involvement. Ketamine was used for fibromyalgia in 2 studies, both showing positive results.

#### 6.4.4 Post amputation/phantom limb pain

This condition is quite resistant to treatment and up to 80% of patients, post amputation, develop phantom pain sometime during their life time. Central sensitization and wind-up phenomenon have been well demonstrated in these conditions. There is reorganisation of cortical representation as well, which is perhaps secondary to the above changes. Ketamine or other NMDA antagonists have a definite role, at least as understood through their pharmacological effects. There have been only 2 studies (Eichenberger, 2008; Nikolajsen, 1996) examining the role of ketamine IV infusions in this condition. Both found positive results with ketamine treatment. Unfortunately the duration of treatment effect has not been clearly followed. Perhaps this condition deserves more studies to establish the role of ketamine in its management.

### 6.4.5 Nerve injury pain and post herpetic neuralgia

These two are considered together as they both involve destruction of nerve elements, and cause deafferentation pain. Altogether there were 4 studies. Gottrup et al (2006) and Jorum et al (2003), both observed a decrease in spontaneous pain and not much effect on allodynia. However, Leung et al (2001) did not find any reduction in spontaneous pain but found decrease in stroking pain score. Eide et al (1994) found a decrease in over all pain score and found no difference in specific pain modalities.

Felsby (1996) used ketamine in peripheral neuropathic pain and found that to significantly benefit spontaneous pain and also touch evoked allodynia.

### 6.4.6 CRPS

3 studies examined the role of ketamine in CRPS. All 3 found positive results. Sigtermans et al (2009) and Dahan et al (2011), both had 60 patients and employed increasing doses of ketamine titrated to best effect. The former study showed statistically significant difference in pain scores between placebo and ketamine, which lasted up to 11 weeks. The latter study employed the same protocol; however the study parameters were different. They performed a pharmacokinetic-pharmacodynamic modeling to study the effect. It demonstrated that the treatment effect/analgesia outlasts the actual treatment period (determined by serum levels) by 50 days. Schwartzman et al (2009) performed an outpatient based ketamine treatment study. Although it planned to include 20 patients in each arm, it was stopped after a total of 19 patients, as the interim analysis showed little placebo effect. CRPS patients showed statistically significant decrease in pain scores over many parameters such as pain the most affected area, burning pain, pain when touched gently, and over all pain score. Follow up to 3 months showed that some treatment effects lasted up to 5-8 weeks (pain when touched). Further they state that the dose employed in that study, 25mg/h (100mg/4h) is perhaps less effective considering their newer treatment protocol using 50mg/h showing much better results. Further studies on larger group of well selected patients are needed to establish the role of ketamine in CRPS.

### 6.4.7 Central pain and spinal cord injury pain

These neuropathic pain conditions are very challenging to treat as they are not localised and involve most parts of the body. The nature of pathology causing pain in these conditions is not clearly known. NMDARs are supposed to play a role. Three studies examined the role of ketamine with spinal cord injury patients. Amr et al (2010) used ketamine with gabapentin and found it to be more effective than gabapentin alone in study of 40 patients. The treatment effect was lost after 3-4 weeks. Kvanstrom et al (2003) used ketamine in a study of 10 patients, with pain below the level of spinal cord injury. Ketamine reduced pain scores >50% in all 5 patients. It is not documented whether there was any longer duration effect. Eide et al (1995) examined 9 patients in a randomised protocol with cross over design. He compared ketamine with alfentanil and a placebo. It was found that both continuous and evoked pains were markedly reduced by the blockade of NMDA receptors by ketamine as well as by the activation of mu-opioid receptors by alfentanil.

| Author/ Year | Design | Patient population and numbers | Design/ Methodology | Outcomes | Withdrawal/ Side Effects |
|---|---|---|---|---|---|
| Amr (2010) | DB RCT PLC | N=40; Neuropathic pain secondary to spinal cord injury | Ketamine (80 mg IV infusion in 500 ml NS over 5 hours) plus 300 mg gabapentin TID vs placebo (NS) and 300 mg gabapentin TID, daily X 1 week | Each day of infusion and weeks 1 and 2 post-infusion treatment arm had lower VAS scores that control arm; effect lost at post-infusion weeks 3 and 4 | 3 patients with short acting delusions after infusion, 2 patients with 15% increase in heart rate during infusion |
| Sitgermans (2009) | SB RCT PLC | N=60; CRPS-1 | Ketamine (1.2 mcg/kg/min IV, increased as tolerated until good pain control up to maximum of 7.2 mcg/kg/min IV) vs Placebo (NS) for 100h | Statistically significant decrease in 10 point pain scale scores up to 12 weeks after initiation of study; no difference in functional improvement | 63% of patients experienced nausea, 47% vomiting, 93% psychomimetic effects |
| Lemming (2007) | DB RCT PLC | N=20; >1 year of whiplash associated pain | Ketamine (IV infused over 20 min to a plasma concentration of 100 ng/ml) vs remifentanil (IV infused over 30 min to a plasma concentration of 1 ng/ml) vs combination vs placebo (NS) x 4 sessions | Both remifentanil and ketamine decreased habitual pain by VAS (no significant difference); ketamine had additional effect on electrical stimulation pain threshold | 15 ketamine only patients experienced some level of sedation, 2 had strange dreams, 1 hallucinations, 1 nausea |
| Lemming (2005) | DB RCT PLC | N=33;Whiplash disorder | Ketamine (0.3 mg/kg IV infused over 30 min) vs Lidocaine (5mg/kg IV) vs morphine (0.3mg/kg IV) vs placebo (NS) x 1 | No significant difference in response between all treatment arms; all treatment arms did illicit partial response | Not Documented |

| Author/ Year | Design | Patient population and numbers | Design/ Methodology | Outcomes | Withdrawal/ Side Effects |
|---|---|---|---|---|---|
| Persson (1998) | DB RCT | N=8; Lower extremity rest pain from arteriosclerosis obliterans | Ketamine (0.15, 0.3, 0.45 mg/kg IV over 2 hr) vs morphine (10 mg IV) x 4 sessions | Dose dependant improvement in resting pain; complete resolution of pain at highest doses | Dose dependent impairment in cognition and perception |
| Yamamoto (1997) | SB RCT PLC | N=39; Central post-stroke pain with thalamic or suprathalamic regions | Ketamine (5mg IV q5min x5) vs Morphine (3mg IV q5min x 6) vs Thiamylal (50mcg IV q5min x 5) vs Placebo (5 ml NS q5min x2) | 47.8% of patients had significant drop in VAS spontaneous pain scores; no comment on significance as compared to other groups | 2 patients had transient hallucinations and anxiety |
| Felsby (1996) | DB RCT PLC | N=10; Neuropathic pain disorders | Ketamine (0.2 mg/kg loading dose followed by 0.3 mg/kg/min infusion for one hour) vs Magnesium Chloride (0.16mmol/kg) vs placebo (NS) | Significant reduction in pain and of area of allodynia by VAS; no change to detection and pain thresholds to mechanical and thermal stimuli | 7 patients reported anxiety or mood symptoms; 2 patients became sedated |
| Max (1995) | DB RCT PLC | N=8; Chronic post-traumatic pain and global allodynia | Ketamine (0.75 mg/kg/hr IV; doubled at 60 and 90 min if no effect, halved if side effects) vs Alfentanil (mean dose 11mg IV) vs placebo (NS) over 2 hours x 1 | Ketamine superior to Alfentanil for peak effect of pain relief and relief of allodynia by VAS pain scores | 3 patients sedated, 2 muteness, 2 dissociative reaction; 2 nausea |
| Backonja (1994) | DB RCT PLC | N=6; Neuropathic pain | Premedicated with benzodiazapine then ketamine (250 mcg/kg IV slow push) vs placebo (NS) | 3/6 patients had at least 50% reduction in pain, 4/6 had similar reduction in allodynia and hyperalgesia | 5 patients had side effects to ketamine (diplopia, nystagmus, psychomimetic effects, increased BP and HR) |

| Author/ Year | Design | Patient population and numbers | Design/ Methodology | Outcomes | Withdrawal/ Side Effects |
|---|---|---|---|---|---|
| Kvarnstron (2004) | 10 PT DB RCT PLC | Spinal Cord Injury with Pain Below Injury Level | Ketamine (0.4 mg/kg IV) vs Lidocaine (2.5 mg/kg IV) vs Placebo (NS) | 5 patients in ketamine group had >50% reduction in spontaneous VAS score 2 hours after administration | 7 patients reported dizziness, changes in vision or somnolence, 5 reported paresthesias |
| Kvarnstrom (2003) | DB RCT PLC | N=12; Long lasting, post-traumatic neuropathic pain | Ketamine (0.4 mg/kg IV) vs Lidocaine (2.5 mg/kg) vs placebo (NS) infused over 40 minutes | Significant improvement in VAS scores with ketamine (mean decrease 55%) compared with placebo; no change in scores of thermal or mechanical stimulation | 100% of subjects reported somnolescence, 75% light-headed, 83% paresthesias, 67% out of body sensation, 50% changes in vision |
| Baad-Hansen (2007) | Case-Control PRO DB PLC | N=20; 10 Patients with atypical odontalgia; 10 healthy age/sex matched controls | Ketamine (50 mcg/kg then 70mcg/kg IV) vs Fentanyl (1.43mcg/kg IV) vs Placebo (NS) | No change in VAS pain score of ongoing AO pain | 5 patients reported dizziness, 4 "feeling drunk", 2 nausea |
| Eide (1994) | DB RCT PLC | N=8; Post-herpetic neuralgia | Ketamine (0.15mg/kg IV) vs morphine vs placebo (NS) | Overall "decrease in pain sensation" and decrease in wind-up pain with ketamine. No significant change in warm, cold, heat or tactile sensation. Both morphine and ketamine improve allodynia compared to placebo; | "Side effects" seen in all 8 ketamine patients |

| Author/ Year | Design | Patient population and numbers | Design/ Methodology | Outcomes | Withdrawal/ Side Effects |
|---|---|---|---|---|---|
| Eide (1995) | DB RCT PLC | N=9; Post spinal cord injury dysethesia | Ketamine (60 mcg/kg bolus then 6 mcg/kg/min) vs alfentanil vs placebo (NS) | Continuous and provoked pain were reduced with ketamine and alfentanil; no change in temperature sensation | "Bothersome dizziness" in one patient |
| Eichenberger et al (2008) | DB PLC RCT | N=20; Phantom limb pain in any extremity from surgical or traumatic amputation | Ketamine (0.4 mg/kg IV over 1 hour with calcitonin 200 IE x 4 total treatments every other day) vs Calcitonin vs placebo vs Ketamine (0.4 mg/kg IV over 1 hour) - later additions to study design | Statistically significant reduction in VAS scores only in ketamine group (not combination). 60% of treatment arm had at least a 50% reduction in symptoms | 5 patients became unconscious, experienced visual hallucination, and hearing impairment during ketamine administration; in combination therapy, 4 patients became nauseous, had visual hallucinations; 9 became dizzy and 1 became unconscious |
| Nikolajsen (1996) | DB RCT PLC | N=11; Post-amputation stump pain | Ketamine (0.1 mg/kg IV bolus then 7 mcg/kg/min over 45 minutes) vs placebo (NS) | Improvement of McGill Pain Questionnaire and VAS pain Scores in treatment arm; decreased incidence of wind-up pain. | 6 patients reported sensation of "insobriety"; 3 reported" discomfort" |
| Sorensen (1997) | DB RCT PLC | N=18; Fibromyalgia | Ketamine (0.3mg/kg IV) vs Morphine (0.3mg/kg IV) vs Lidocaine (5mg/kg IV) vs Placebo (NS) x 1 dose | All treatment arms showed significant reduction of resting pain; no comment on superiority/ inferiority of ketamine to other treatments | Not Documented |

| Author/ Year | Design | Patient population and numbers | Design/ Methodology | Outcomes | Withdrawal/ Side Effects |
|---|---|---|---|---|---|
| Graven-Nielsen (2000) | DB RCT PLC | N=29; Fibromyalgia | Ketamine (0.3 mg/kg) vs placebo (NS) over 30 minutes over 2 separate days [ketamine sensitivity detection]; ketamine vs placebo (NS) over 2 separate days with one week washout [ketamine effect] | Decrease in VAS score during and up to 60 minutes after infusion; decrease in referred pain and temporal pain | Not documented |
| Leung (2001) | DB RCT PLC | N=12; Post nerve damage pain | ketamine (IV infusion targeted to 50, 100 and 150 ng/ml) vs alfentanil (IV infusion targeted to 25, 50 and 75 ng/ml) vs placebo (diphenhydrinate) | No reduction in spontaneous VAS pain scores; dose dependant decrease in stroking pain score. | 1/3 of ketamine subjects reported light-headedness, 3 subjects sedated |
| Mitchell (2002) | DB PLC RCT | N=35; Alloynia, hyperalgesi a and hyperpathia secondary to critical limb ischemia | Ketamine (0.6 mg/m IV) with normal opioid doses vs placebo (NS) over 4 hours | 69% of patients reported BPI improvement 5 days post administration | 6 patients "felt more emotional than usual" |
| Gottrup (2006) | DB RCT PLC | N=19; Patients with nerve damage and allodynia | Ketamine (0.1 mg/kg IV bolus, then 0.007 mg/kg/min infusion over 7 minutes) vs lidocaine (5mg/kg IV) vs placebo (NS) | Reduction of spontaneous pain by VAS (mean 30% reduction), reduction of evoked pain to brush and pinprick by electronic VAS. No effect on allodynia. | 5 patients reported tiredness, 4 dizziness, 4 paresthesia, 3 dry mouth, 1 patient dropped from study for aggressive behaviour and hallucinations |

| Author/ Year | Design | Patient population and numbers | Design/ Methodology | Outcomes | Withdrawal/ Side Effects |
|---|---|---|---|---|---|
| Schwartzman (2009) | DB RCT PLC | N=19; At least 6 mo of CRPS and failed three previous treatments | 0.1 mg Clonidine and 2 mg of Midazolam then Ketamine (0.35 mg/kg infusion over 4 hours; 50% first day 75% second day) vs placebo (NS) | Statistically significant decrease in 'pain in most affected area', 'burning pain' 'overall pain; and 'pain when lightly touched' by pain questionnaire; ketamine group did not return to baseline level of pain | 4 people in ketamine group reported nausea, headache, tiredness or dysphoria |
| Mercadante (2000) | DB RCT PLC | N=10; Cancer patients on morphine therapy and Karnofsky score > 50 | Ketamine (0.25 mg/kg) vs ketamine (0.5mg/kg) vs placebo (NS) infused over 30 minutes x 1 each | Significant decrease in pain intensity at both ketamine doses 3 hours after administration on 10 point scale; more pronounced with 0.5mg/kg dose | 4 patients experienced hallucinations; 2 patients experienced "out-of-body" sensation |
| Jorum (2003) | DB RCT PLC | N=12; Post traumatic or herpetic neuralgia | Ketamine (60 mcg/kg over 5 min then 6 mcg/kg/min for 20 min) vs alfentanil (7 mcg/kg bolus then 0.6 mcg/kg/min for 20 min) vs placebo (NS) x 1 session each | Decrease in VAS score to spontaneous pain and thermal hyperalgesia; no change on thermal cold threshold | 5 patients experienced fatigue, 6 experienced dizziness, 3 experienced "feeling of unreality", 8 patients reported feeling intoxicated/ relaxed |
| Oga (2002) | SB RCT PLC | N=10; Chronic neuropathic pain | Placebo (5ml NS IV) x 2 then Ketamine (5 mg IV q5min) x 3 | Average decrease on NRS pain scale from 10 to 3.75 with ketamine treatment compared with no significant decrease in saline treatment | Overall significant increase in BRPS scale of negative symptoms (blunted affect, emotional withdrawal and motor retardation) |

Table 5. RCTs of IV Route

## 7. IV ketamine regimen

In experimental ischemic pain, it was observed that there were consistent increases of pain thresholds for plasma concentrations of racemic ketamine more than 160 ng/mL (0.36 µmol/L) (Clements, 1982). However, it has been difficult to establish clear dose-response relationship in clinical situations. The solution used for anesthesia is also utilised to prepare appropriate solutions for parenteral infusions. When given as an infusion, it can be diluted with NS (normal saline 0.9%) in a 1:1 strength (100 mg ketamine in 100 ml NS), and infused via a infusor for accuracy. The administration of ketamine must happen on a fully monitored place with appropriate resuscitation equipments.

As a general statement, parenteral administration, IV or SC, in the range 0.125–0.5 mg/kg/hr, appears to be optimal (level II) but there are occasional reports of larger or smaller doses (Hocking, 2003). The titration is usually dictated by patient's tolerability and clinical usefulness. Frequent (30 mins to 60 mins) assessments of pain and other measures of analgesia must be done. Once a reasonable upper level of infusion is established it may be given for 2-3 days. However there are no clear recommendations, but anecdotal reports suggest that a longer duration of treatment has more chance of effective analgesic actions which are prolonged and sustained. We have observed that the effects in some patients might last up to weeks to months.

If intermittent dosing is planned, it may be wise to consider night-time dosing as it can reduce side effects (level IV), perhaps because of the fact that patients tend to be more relaxed or perhaps because sleep intervenes (Hocking, 2003).

## 8. Conversion to oral ketamine (initiation and maintenance)

In opioid naïve patients, the recommended starting dosage in ketamine naïve patients is 0.5 mg/kg racemic ketamine or 0.25 mg/kg S-ketamine as a single oral dose. Doses can be increased in steps of 0.5 or 0.25 mg/kg according to the efficacy and adverse effects, respectively (Blonk, 2010).

According to Soto et al (2011), oral ketamine seems to be most effective when used at an initial dose of 0.3 to 0.7 mg/kg per d, titrated up to every 6 hours. This is based on several case reports most of which have used an initial parenteral test. For use of oral ketamine at the end of life, data published suggests a starting dose of 30 to 150 mg/d titrated up to 60 to 375 mg/d as the final dose.

For patients who have been on parenteral ketamine, the dose conversion is not simple. Blonk suggests that the daily dosage can be kept equal and, depending on clinical effect and/or adverse effects, is slowly increased (Blonk 2010). This is mostly in contrast with others who recommend lower conversion rates. Fitzgibbon and others started with a lower dose which was approximately one-third of the parenteral ketamine dose (Fitzgibbon, 2002). Most agree that a conversion factor of 15% is appropriate (Soto, 2011). Convert from intravenous to oral route using at least 15% of the total parenteral dose in up to 4 divided doses (70-kg patient, intravenous ketamine infusion 0.1mg/kg per h ¼ oral ketamine 20 mg every 12 hours). After the intravenous infusion, reduce opiate by 25% daily, once adequate analgesia has been reached. Titrate up by 0.3 mg/kg daily until adequate analgesia is achieved or side effects occur. The number of divided doses necessary for continuous analgesic effect can range from once daily up to a frequency of 6 times daily (Blonk 2010). The duration of effect after a single dose can range from a few hours to 24 h or more.

## 9. Challenges and limitations of ketamine use in chronic pain

1. Unavailability: the use of Ketamine for chronic pain is not approved and is off label. There are no commercially available preparations. The injection solution has been used, both for parenteral and oral use. Because of its higher potency, the S (+) racemate of ketamine is approved for use in Europe where it is commercially available as a preservative-free formulation for the treatment of pain by oral, parenteral, and neuroaxial administration (Ben Ari, 2007).
2. Choosing the right patient, in terms of responsiveness.
3. Choosing the right dose, duration and route of administration: There are no fixed strategies. Even if a patient is responsive to parenteral ketamine he may not be as responsive in the longer run (Hocking, 2003). For oral route, the dose conversion is not straight forward and not based solely on decreased bioavailability.
4. There is no consistent dose-response relation. Even if one theoretically takes the serum levels of ketamine to maintain it at only a level required for therapeutic actions and not unwanted side effects, it is not possible to do so as the pharmacodynamics is still not entirely clear.
5. Managing side effects; specific side effects related to subcutaneous and intranasal route have been mentioned above. The most frequently observed adverse effects were effects on the central nervous system, such as sedation, somnolence, dizziness, sensory illusions, hallucinations, nightmares, dissociative feeling and blurred vision. Most consider hallucinations as most disturbing (Blonk, 2010). Patients also mentioned gastrointestinal adverse effects, such as nausea, vomiting, anorexia and abdominal pain. It is also known to cystitis and other urinary complications when used on a longer duration and in addicts.
6. Addiction: It is used as a street drug because of its psychotomimetic properties. It can be obtained as powder by heating the injection fluid, and used through snorting or inhaling (Blonk, 2010).
7. Monitoring for long term effects and change: Long term effects are unknown. There have been only a few case reports which have followed the patients for months to years on ketamine treatment. The knowledge that NMDA receptors are associated with several other functions, it is prudent to assume that long term side effects are possible, and should be kept in mind.

## 10. Long term use

In neuropathic pain patients on long term treatment, Enarson (1999) used oral ketamine up to 100-240 mg per day in 14% patients who continued to use it for at least an year. Many others have used it on a long term basis (Furuhashi-Yonaha, 2002). Lack of evidence regarding efficacy, and the poor safety profile, do not support routine use of oral ketamine in chronic pain management. There is only one case series (N = 32) which specifically studied the side-effects of ketamine in the long-term treatment (3 months) of neuropathic pain (Cvrcek P, 2008). Literature is not conclusive about the differences in safety profiles of ketamine as racemic mixture and S-ketamine (Kohrs, 1998).

## 11. Conclusions

Since there are no guidelines or good evidence regarding the introduction and use of ketamine in chronic pain conditions, the above based indications are mostly based on clinical reasoning, mostly with the view that NMDA receptors are involved in the generation or sustenance of the pain condition. Chronic pain conditions are quite heterogeneous in their pathophysiology; and there is still a huge knowledge gap in understanding several of them with regards to their clinical symptoms and variations. We also do not know how ketamine modulates pain pathways or its various actions leading to analgesic mechanisms. We still do not know whether oral route is better for analgesia. It has been suggested that oral ketamine administration causes fewer side effects (Hocking, 2003). Perhaps because of the smaller plasma levels an improved side effect profile of nor-ketamine is observed. With the above considerations, we are left with exploring its analgesic potential for the benefit of patients who have resistant chronic pain condition, despite not so good evidence. Many to most patients do not respond; in fact according to some estimates only up to 30% respond (Hocking, 2003). Considering placebo responses come quite close to it in numbers, it is not certain if it's a true response. Rabben and Oye suggested that there could be changes which may make the patient not susceptible to NMDA antagonists, as the clinical condition worsens. We might be able to improve the numbers of true responders if we get to know whether there are any variables, either disease specific or patient specific, telling us which patients may respond. In that direction there has to be further research and exploration. Until then it is not easy to formulate evidence based guidelines, despite having so many RCTs. From a present stand point use of ketamine is still directed by personal/clinician's preference, availability of resources, patient's acceptability, and above all a patient specific approach in terms of appropriate route, dose and duration.

## Part B: Lidocaine

## 12. Pharmacological basis of Lidocaine use in neuropathic pain

Lidocaine is a local anesthetic compound belonging to the amide group. The chemical structure of lidocaine is 2,6-xylidine coupled to diethylglycine by an amide bond. Lidocaine was first synthesized in 1943 and was used for many years as a local anesthetic agent. It is metabolized chiefly by the liver, and the major pathway of degradation involves conversion to monoethylglycylxylidide, to 2,6-xylidine and finally to 4-hydroxy-2,6-xylidine. These and various other metabolites are excreted in the urine. In addition, a small percentage of unchanged lidocaine, up to 10 percent, is also excreted in the urine.The major metabolic end product is 4-hydroxy-2,6-xylidine since up to 70 percent of an administered dose of lidocaine appears as this compound in the urine. The chemical structure of lidocaine is given as below.

Lidocaine has been well studied and used as a local anesthetic agent. It was realised to have antiarrhythmic potential and has also been widely used for that purpose, as class IB agent. The first clinical use of lidocaine infusion in pain treatments was by 2 anesthesiologists (Bartlett and Hutaserani, 1961), for post-operative pain relief. Since then it has been used for various chronic pain syndromes, mostly of neuropathic nature, such as diabetic neuropathy, postherpetic neuralgia, and deafferentation pain.

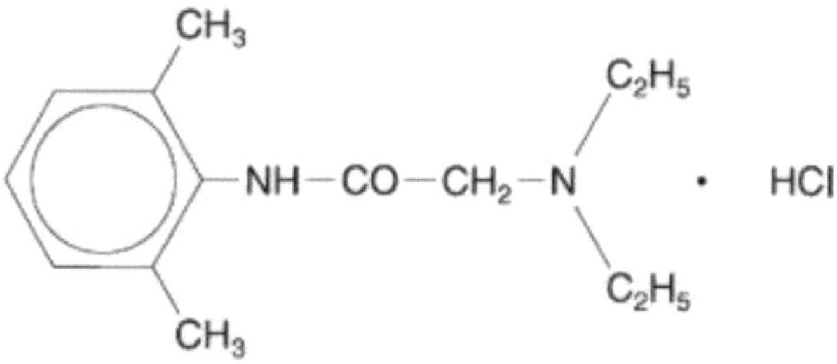


Fig. 3. Lidocaine chemical structure

How exactly systemic lidocaine works in neuropathic pain conditions and why it does work on only a selected number of patients is not yet completely known. However, the following description is based on the presently accepted concept (Mao & Chen, 2000).

1. Lidocaine acts on sodium channel receptors which functions as the basic unit of nerve action potential generation.
2. Neuropathic pain generates from ectopic, abnormal discharges of injured nerves in many neuropathic pain conditions (Nordin 1984).
3. Lidocaine is supposed to have a differential action; suppresses the ectopic discharges but does not interfere in the normal neural discharges.

Neuropathic pain is complex and heterogeneous. Apart from various diverse etiologies, it is also suggested that within diagnostic groups of neuropathic pain patients, there may be subgroups with distinct mechanisms and therefore possibly differing responses to drug treatments (Attal, 2004). Symptoms and signs of neuropathic pain may include spontaneous pain, hyperalgesia, allodynia, pain summation, and radiation of pain beyond the affected area (Dyke, 1984).There are many animal studies indicating that peripheral mechanisms of neuropathic pain may involve spontaneous ectopic discharges from the injured nerves. Experimentally, such injury may involve the form of complete deafferentation, loose nerve ligation, ligation of individual nerve root (Mao & Chen, 2000). When a peripheral nerve is injured the afferent input can be generated spontaneously without activation of peripheral receptors. Such input is referred to as spontaneous ectopic discharges (Devor, 1991). Electrophysiological studies have suggested that ectopic discharges can be initiated along the injured nerve, DRG, and peripheral neuromata (Wall and Gutnick, 1974; Mao & Chen, 2000). Such ectopic discharges may last for a few hours to many days after nerve injury. It is possible to distinguish the origin of ectopic discharges as "neuromata- high frequency, rhythmic, spontaneous discharges" and "DRG neurons- slow, irregular activities in the absence of central or peripheral input". Such aberrant, ectopic action potentials are supposed to be conducted along the nerve via the activation of sodium channels.

## 13. Sodium channel and neuropathic pain

The voltage-gated ion channels (VGICs) are a super family of glycoprotein molecules that form membrane spanning channels that 'gate' in response to changes in membrane potential. The biophysical properties include: channel opening or 'activation' which is dependent upon membrane potential, rapid 'inactivation' (which is governed not only by membrane potential but also time) and selective ion conductance. The major structural component of the channel is a protein of approximately 260 kDa that has been named the alpha subunit. The alpha subunit comprises four repeated structural motifs (named I–IV) consisting of six alpha helical transmembrane spanning domains separated by intra and extracellular loops. These four repeated domains fold together to form a central pore and it is their structural components that determine selectivity and conductance of the ion (Scolz A, 2002). The central pore has been determined to be aqueous in nature as it has the capacity to conduct very large numbers of sodium ions through a single channel. By electrophysiology, biochemical purification and cloning, several different sodium channel a-subunits, named as "NaV1.1–1.9" have been identified. Studies have shown a link between several Nav channels and pain, namely 1.3, 1.7, 1.8 and 1.9. Nav 1.3 mediates the compound tetrodotoxin (TTX), a poison from the puffer fish, and has faster activation and inactivation kinetics. It is highly expressed in sensory nerve tracts and spinal cord white matter, dorsal roots and deep laminae of the dorsal and ventral horn. This channel is supposed to be involved in the development of spontaneous ectopic discharges and sustained firing associated with the injured nerves. Nav 1.3 expression is seen to be increased 20-30 fold in neuropathic pain models. Nav 1.7 and Nav 1.9 are observed to be associated with inflammatory or nociceptive pain (Wood et al, 2004). Functionally the sodium channels exist in three possible conformational states and it is the transition between these states that allows selective and temporally regulated ionic conductance. When a stimulus provides a depolarizing change in the cellular membrane potential, the ion channels undergo a physical conformational change and the so-called 'activation gate' is opened. Activation is very rapid, occurring within a fraction of a millisecond and is due to movement of gating charges within the membrane electric field. When the activation gate is opened, the channel pore selectively conducts sodium ions down an electrochemical gradient from the extracellular space to the cell interior. Within a few milliseconds, the sustained depolarization results in termination of the sodium conductance by a process known as inactivation. This occurs very

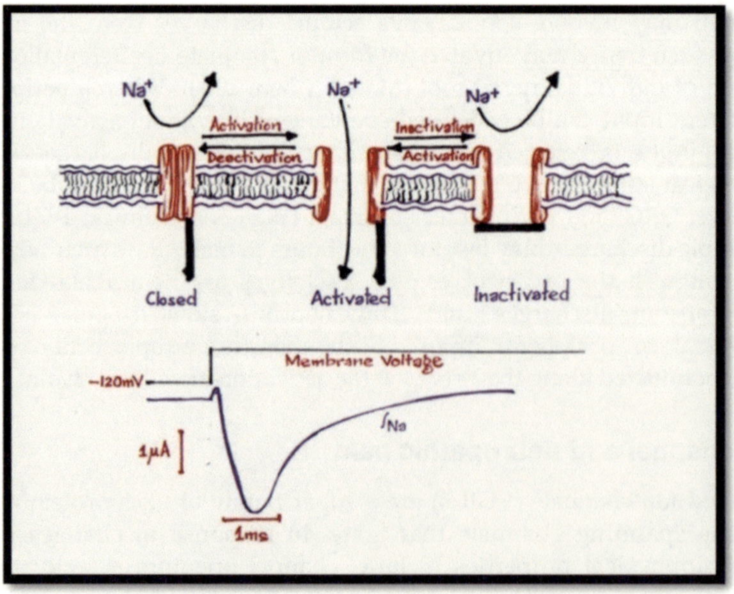


Fig. 4. Sodium channel kinetics as related to membrane potential

rapidly, producing attenuation of the sodium current and for this reason the process is often referred to as 'fast' inactivation. The second type of sodium channel inactivation, termed slow, occurs next. The ability of channels to recover from the fast inactivated state is dependent upon membrane potential and time, and is a mechanism that ensures adequate time for recovery before reopening of the channel.

Local anesthetics, including lidocaine are charged at a $P_H$ below 6. The uncharged form is lipid soluble. It is now well understood and appreciated that LAs diffuse across the lipid membrane before getting to their active site. The receptor lies within the pore. The charged form of the compound acts on the receptor in a use dependent or phasic block. This means increasing impulses leads to accumulation of inhibition. The guarded hypothesis theory also means the binding site is within the pore and the pore has to be open for the LA molecule to bind. The impact of use dependent block would mean that as the firing frequency of the nerve fibre increases, lower concentrations of local anesthetics would be needed to block the action potentials (Scholz A, 2002).

## 14. Lidocaine in neuropathic pain

Lidocaine acts on these sodium channels to block the impulse transmission and selectively act on ectopic discharges (spontaneously produced without external stimuli). It is not clear, however, whether LAs acts by blocking impulse propagation or whether it prevents the very initiation of abnormal discharge. This should lead to the clinical inference that spontaneous pain symptoms must be more susceptible for lidocaine induced pain relief rather than evoked pain symptoms. In human studies on neuromata, two studies examined spontaneous discharges associated with peripheral nerve fibres following limb amputation. Spontaneous nerve activities recorded were not changed after local infiltration of neuromata with 1% lidocaine indicating a source of generators independent of neuromata. However, local lidocaine does block burst activities induced by tapping neuromata (Mao & Chen, 2000). However this is not the case in many other studies. On further analysis, it is also proposed that allodynia may represent a central phenomenon which is secondarily activated because of the sensitization of sodium channels on Ab fibres. In this regard, a model of neuropathic pain has been proposed in which ongoing nociceptive afferent input from a peripheral locus is thought to maintain the dynamically-altered central process underlying allodynia (Mao & Chen, 2000).

1. **Acting peripherally**, a number of studies have demonstrated that lidocaine suppresses ectopic activity arising out of injured neurons at clinically relevant doses. Another interesting observation is that systemic lidocaine has been shown to have dissociative effects on nerve conduction and ectopic discharges, i.e. suppression of ectopic discharges without blocking nerve conduction (Devor et al, 1992), indicating that sodium channels generating ectopic discharges are likely to be different from those mediating normal action potential conduction along a peripheral nerve.
2. **At the level of spinal cord**, lidocaine is also known to induce a selective depression of C fibre-evoked activity among spinal cord-wide dynamic range neurons and decrease the hyperexcitability of dorsal horn neurons in neuropathic pain models (Woolf, 1985).
3. **Supraspinal** mechanisms of lidocaine actions are demonstrated by its effectiveness in hemispheric lesions and central pain (Attal et al, 2000). Lidocaine can also induce changes in neuropathic pain behaviours (Mao & Chen, 2000). Neuropathic pain

behaviours responding to systemic lidocaine include hyperalgesia and allodynia. Procaine infusions on healthy volunteers have shown selective activation of anterior amygdalocentric limbic system. Lidocaine infusions can give rise to acute psychiatric reactions especially in patients having significant affective component (Leong & Solason, 2000).

## 15. Lidocaine use in clinical practice

Clinically the response to lidocaine varies in different chronic pain syndromes. In general peripheral neuropathic conditions are more susceptible (Galer et al, 1993; Tremont-Lukats et al, 2005; Attal et al, 2000). Even with the same condition the responsiveness may differ between two individuals with similar history and symptoms. Further even in a single patient only a subset of neuropathic pain symptoms (modality specific) may be responsive. Using quantitative sensory tests, Attal et al have shown that IV lidocaine induced selective and differential analgesic effects in patients with central neuropathic pain (Attal et al, 2000). Ketamine alleviated spontaneous pain and mechanical allodynia/hyperalgesia, but had no effect on thermal allodynia/hyperalgesia. Wallace et al studied the effects of IV lidocaine in CRPS patients and used diphenhydramine as a control. Intravenous lidocaine and diphenhydramine had no significant effect on the cool, warm, or cold pain thresholds. The effect on allodynia was seen only at the maximum plasma range. Lidocaine affected pain in response to cool stimuli more than mechanical pain in subjects with neuropathic pain (Wallace et al, 2000). This is in contrast to the study by Attal et al. Hence it is still not certain which modalities of neuropathic pain are particularly sensitive to lidocaine infusions.

Previously lidocaine was given as IV boluses; presently it is mostly given as an infusion. In many centres it is given using a computer controlled, targeted infusions. The commonly used range is 3-5mg/kg over 30-60 minutes. This may or may not involve an initial bolus. Most studies have shown to achieve a plasma concentration of 2-5 μg/ml (Mao & Chen, 2000). Ferrante et al studied the dose response and plasma concentration in 13 patients. Lidocaine was given at a rate of 8.35 mg/min (500 mg). Ten patients had complete pain relief as measured by VAS scores and scores from the short form of the McGill Pain Questionnaire and the Multidimensional Pain Inventory. After a certain plasma level of 0.62 μg/ml, there were steep changes of pain scores with small changes in lidocaine plasma concentration (Ferrante 1996). Carroll et al employed an appropriate dose to produce plasma levels of 5 μg/ml (Carroll 2007). Indeed up to 15 μg/ml was achieved in some initial studies without serious sequelae (Schinder, 1996; Carroll, 2007). Not much knowledge is available regarding the duration of pain relief after an IV bolus versus continuous infusion of lidocaine. The onset of lidocaine effect on pain relief ranges from 1 to 45 min after lidocaine administration (Mao & Chen, 2000; Carroll, 2007). There is still no consensus about the appropriate duration of observation after either lidocaine bolus or infusion. Apart from the anecdotal reports there are no studies documenting longer lasting pain relief (days-months).

## 16. Review of literature

The use of lidocaine in clinical practice has been well reviewed earlier by Tremont-Lukats et al (Tremont-Lukats et al, 2005). Their systematic search revealed 13 trials using lidocaine infusion. Most of these studies have fewer subjects and tend to suffer from the fallacy of

| Study | Design | Patient Population | Treatment | Outcomes | Adverse/Side Effects |
|---|---|---|---|---|---|
| Gottrup (2006) | DB RCT PLC | N=19, Patients with nerve damage and allodynia | Ketamine (0.1 mg/kg IV bolus, then 0.007 mg/kg/min infusion over 7 minutes) vs lidocaine (5mg/kg IV over 30 min) vs placebo (NS) | Both ketamine and lidocaine significantly reduced evoked pain to pinprick stimuli; ketamine was superior to lidocaine in reducing spontaneous pain | 7 tiredness, 4 nausea, 3 paresthesia, 3 blurred vision, 3 changed taste, 3 dysarthria, 2 headache, 2 dry mouth |
| Viola (2006) | DB RCT PLC | N=15, diabetic neuropathy, previous responders to lidocaine | Lidocaine (5mg/ml IV) vs Lidocaine (7.5mg/ml IV) vs placebo (NS), 5ml/kg over 4 hours x 1 each, four week washout | Both doses of lidocaine decreased MPQ resting pain scores compared to placebo; effect lasted up to 28 days post-infusion | 1 patient reported light-headedness with 7.5 mg/ml infusion |
| Finnerup (2005) | DB RCT PLC | N=24, spinal cord injury with neuralgia at or below level of injury | Lidocaine (5mg/kg IV) vs placebo (NS) over 30 min x 1 | Significant reduction of spontaneous pain in treatment group; no effect on evoked pain | 11 somnolence, 7 dizziness, 7 dysarthria, 7 lightheaded, 3 blurred vision |
| Attal (2004) | DB RCT PLC | N=22, post-herpatic or post-traumatic neuralgia | Lidocaine (5mg/kg IV) vs placebo (NS) over 30 min x1 | Significant reduction of spontaneous pain by VAS, as well as mechanical allodynia; no effect on thermal or hyperalgesia | 16 patients experienced side effects including somnolence, lightheadedness, periorbital numbness |
| Medrik-Goldberg (1999) | DB RCT PLC | N=30, Sciatica | Lidocaine (5mg/kg IV) vs amantadine (2.5mg/kg IV) vs placebo (NS) over 2 hours x 1 | Lidocaine significantly reduced spontaneous pain on VAS scale up to 30 min after infusion as compared with amantadine and placebo; also significant decrease in SLR evoked pain compared to other two arms | None reported |

| Study | Design | Patient Population | Treatment | Outcomes | Adverse/Side Effects |
|---|---|---|---|---|---|
| Scrivani (1999) | SB RCT PLC | N=30, Chronic neurogenic facial pain | Lidocaine (100mg IV) vs Phentolamine (30mg IV) vs placebo (NS) infused over 5-10 min x 1 | Lidocaine infusion decreased spontaneous pain in 16 patient on 10 point VAS for up to 30 min | None reported |
| Baranowsky (1999) | DB RCT PLC | N=24, post-herpatic neuralgia | Lidocaine (0.5 mg/kg/h IV) vs Lidocaine (2.5mg/kg/h IV) vs placebo (NS) over 2 hours x 1 | No significant difference in spontaneous pain on MCQ and VAS pain scales, allodynia and pressure provoked pain were both significantly improved with either dose of lidocaine | Not reported |
| Galer (1996) | DB RCT | N=9, Peripheral neuropathic pain | Lidocaine (2mg/kg IV) vs Lidocaine (5 mg/kg IV) over 45 min x 1 | Both arms had significant decrease in VAS resting pain scores; higher dose lidocaine produced significantly greater pain relief than lower dose | 1 patient dropped out due to severe dizziness and tinnitus |
| Wallace (1996) | DB RCT PLC | N=11, post-traumatic neuropathic pain | Lidocaine (targeted plasma concentrations of 0.5, 1, 1.5, 2 and 2.5 mcg/ml sustained over 10 min) vs placebo (NS) x 1 each | Significant decrease in spontaneous VAS pain scores starting at 1.5mcg/ml concentration; no change in evoked pain | 6 patients reported lightheadednes s, 1 patient reported nausea |
| Bruera (1992) | DB RCT PLC | N=?, Neuropathic cancer pain | Lidocaine (5mg/kg IV) vs Placebo (NS) over 30 min x 1 | No change in VAS pain scores between groups | Unknown |
| Rowbotham (1991) | DB RCT PLC | N=19, Post-herpetic neuralgia | Lidocaine (?IV) vs Morphine (?IV) vs Placebo (NS) | Both morphine and lidocaine reduced pain intensity | Unknown |

| Study | Design | Patient Population | Treatment | Outcomes | Adverse/Side Effects |
|---|---|---|---|---|---|
| Wallace (2000) | DB RCT PLC | N=16, CRPS 1 and 2 | Lidocaine (1,2,3mcg/ml plasma IV) vs placebo (diphenhydramine) x 1 | Significant decrease in spontaneous VAS pain scores in 3mcg/ml; all concentrations caused significant decrease in response to stroking and cool stimuli in the affected area | Average side effect score (out of 100) for light headedness and sedation was more significant than placebo |
| Ellemann (1989) | DB RCT PLC | N=10, Cancer patients with cutaneous allodynia | Lidocaine (5mg/kg IV) vs placebo (NS) x 1 | 2 patients reported subjective pain relief in treatment arm, 3 in placebo arm | Unknown |
| Sharma (2009) | DB RCT PLC | N=50, cancer patients with opioid refractory pain | Lidocaine (2mg/kg bolus over 20 minutes followed by 2mg/kg infusion over 2 hr) vs placebo (NS) | Significant decrease in 10 point numeric pain scores in treatment group after 2 hours; significantly longer duration of analgesia than placebo | 7 patients with periorbital numbness, 8 with tinnitus |
| Kastrup (1987) | DB RCT PLC | N=?, Diabetic neuropathy of >6 months | Lidocaine (5mg/kg IV) vs placebo (NS) | Significant beneficial effect of lidocaine arm on pain symptoms 1 and 8 days post infusion | Unknown |
| Tremonts-Lukats (2006) | DB RCT PLC | N=32, Peripheral neuropathic pain | Lidocaine (1,3,5 mg/kg IV) vs placebo (NS) over 6 hours x 1 each | Significant change in percentage pain intensity difference between 5mg/kg arm and placebo up to four hours post-infusion | 10 light-headedness, 4 nausea, 6 periorbial numbness, 6 headache, 3 incoordination |
| Gormsen (2009) | DB RCT PLC | N=13, chronic neuropathic pain | Lidocaine (5mg/kg IV) vs NS1209 (AMPA receptor antagonist 322 mg total) vs placebo (NS) over 4 hours x1 | No difference in any treatment arms of spontaneous current pain, both NS1209 and lidocaine exhibited significant effects on resting pain compared to placebo | All lidocaine patients experienced adverse events including headache, dizziness, somnolence, fatigue, cognitive impairment |

| Study | Design | Patient Population | Treatment | Outcomes | Adverse/Side Effects |
|---|---|---|---|---|---|
| Attal (2000) | DB RCT PLC | N=16, post stroke or spinal cord injury pain | Lidocaine (5mg/kg IV) vs placebo (NS) over 30 min x 1 | Significant reduction in spontaneous pain on VAS in treatment arm; no significant difference in mechanical or thermal stimulation thresholds | 7 patients with light-headedness, 5 somnolence, 3 nausea/ vomiting, 3 dysarthria, 2 malaise |
| Marchettni (1992) | RCT PLC | N=10, organic nerve injury causing neuropathic pain | Lidocaine (unknown IV) vs Placebo (NS) | Subjective report of mechanical hyperalgesia and spontaneous pain decreased significantly in treatment arm | Unknown |
| Wu (2002) | DB PLC RCT | N=32, phantom limb or stump pain | Lidocaine (1mg/kg bolus then 4mg/kg IV) vs Morphine (0.05mg/kg bolus then 0.2mg/kg IV) vs placebo (Diphenhydramine 10mg bolus then 40 mg IV) over 40 min x 1 | Lidocaine significantly decreased stump pain by VAS pain score, Morphine decreased both stump and phantom limb pain. | No difference in sedation scores between treatment arms |
| Kvarnstrom (2003) | 12 PT DB RCT PLC | Long lasting, post-traumatic neuropathic pain | Ketamine (0.4 mg/kg IV) vs Lidocaine (2.5 mg/kg) vs placebo (NS) infused over 40 minutes | No significant difference in VAS resting score between lidocaine and placebo; no significant difference in any evoked VAS scores | 9 somnolence, 5 light-headedness, 4 "out of body sensation", 3 nausea, 2 pruritis, 2 paresthesia |
| Kvarnstron (2004) | 10 PT DB RCT PLC | Spinal Cord Injury with Pain Below Injury Level | Ketamine (0.4 mg/kg IV) vs Lidocaine (2.5 mg/kg IV) vs Placebo (NS) over 40 min | No significant difference in response between lidocaine and placebo in VAS spontaneous pain scores and evoked allodynia | 5 somnolence, 1 dizziness, 2 out of body sensation, 1 change in hearing, 2 paresthesias |
| Lemming (2005) | 33 PT DB RCT PLC | Patients with whiplash disorder | Ketamine (0.3 mg/kg infused over 30 min) vs Lidocaine vs morphine vs placebo (NS) | No significant difference in response between all treatment arms; all treatment arms did illicit partial response | Not Documented |

Table 6. RCTs of IV Lidocaine use

heterogeneity with respect to disease treated, dose employed and outcomes measured. Despite the deficiencies, they were able to synthesise the data and do a meta-analysis. For the lidocaine trials considered for analysis, the median Jadad score was 3. In the lidocaine trials included for meta-analysis 165 patients received lidocaine and 164 patients were treated with placebo. Lidocaine was superior to placebo (Weighted Mean Difference -10.02 mm; 95% CI: -16.51 to -3.54 mm, $P > 0.002$). The study concluded that systemic administration of sodium channel blocking drugs can relieve pain in selected patients with neuropathic pain and that this effect is superior to placebo. However, the mean effect was small (approximately 11 mm point on a 100 point scale). The commonly used dose range of lidocaine was 5mg/kg over 30-60 mins. The therapeutic benefit was seen more consistently with peripheral pain-trauma, diabetes and central pain. The duration of pain relief observed with lidocaine infusions are mostly short lived (up to 24 hrs). The same conclusion was drawn in the meta-analysis. Some animal experiments and few human trials have demonstrated prolonged effects far beyond the beyond the pharmacological half-time of lidocaine (Mao & Chen, 2000; Chaplan et al, 1995; Sinnott et al, 1999). The mechanism behind this is unknown.

Another important drawback of most studies was the outcome measures considered; allodynia which is an evoked pain measure rather than spontaneous pain was evaluated. This study has also been criticized as the conclusions may not be clinically relevant, however good methodology has been employed. Because of the quality of the studies the calculation of side effects was significantly affected resulting in inappropriate conclusions (Rathmell & Ballantyne, 2005). Our search identified 23 studies and was further cross referenced with the studies in the systematic review. The table gives a complete list of studies including methodology, results and complications. The place of IV lidocaine infusion in treating neuropathic pain patients is difficult to establish. In clinical practice it may be looked as an additional tool for diagnosis and therapeutic management, mostly to be used in resistant or challenging neuropathic pain conditions when other treatments fail. It could also be used to provide relief in "acute on chronic pain" conditions. Some use an algorithm in which an IV therapeutic drug is utilised only after testing the patient with 1-2 placebo treatments. But most employ a lidocaine test (see below), where in the patient is tested for responsiveness with increasing doses of lidocaine.

## 17. Intravenous lidocaine test

This is a test done to observe for pain relief achieved with IV lidocaine infusion. This is called a test only, because it is the first time that a particular patient having a specific neuropathic pain is being exposed to this treatment. Unlike a known analgesic such as opioid, lidocaine may not be effective or may cause significant dose related side effects even at minimal therapeutic range, which would limit its role in further management of pain condition. Since the effects are immediate and do not take time, one can quickly establish the clinical usefulness in a particular patient.

This is done in an appropriately monitored setting including heart rate, ECG, blood pressure and pulse oximetry. In fact, there are no strict or established protocols. These variations make the usefulness of this test individual specific and generalisations cannot be made. The dose range of systemic lidocaine in the test varies extensively among pain centers, from 100 mg/patient to 5 mg/kg of a patient's body weight (Mao & Chen 2000). The rate of administration also varies from an IV push to a slow infusion over 30-60 min. Similarly the outcome measures of the lidocaine test also differ among pain centers: (1) what to measure to determine a positive test result, (2) how much change to be expected to indicate a positive result, and (3) when to measure after the lidocaine test to determine the test results. Some centres do blinding as reported earlier, however the blinding itself can be questioned as there are no active placebo controls. It is practically impossible for a patient not to notice CNS side-effects after systemic lidocaine administration. Wallace et al used diphenhydramine as a placebo in their study (Wallace et al, 2000). This is perhaps appropriate considering its side effect as a sedative and causing light headedness, similar to lidocaine.

## 18. Lidocaine test for the diagnosis of neuropathic pain syndromes

Perhaps the lidocaine test has more value as a diagnostic tool to identify true neuropathic pain patients rather than a prognosticator for further lidocaine treatment. Marchettini performed this test on ten patients with organic nerve injury causing chronic neuropathic pain. The effect of intravenous lidocaine versus saline was tested using psychophysical somatosensory variables. The variables assessed were the subjective magnitude of pain, area of mechanical hyperalgesia and presence and magnitude of thermal heat/cold hyperalgesia. Lidocaine was given in a dose of 1.5mg/kg over 60 secs and placebo-saline in the other group. The patients were then tested at 5, 15 and 35 mins intervals. It was found that spontaneous pain and mechanical hyperalgesia were consistently improved, transiently, by intravenous administration of lidocaine in all 10 patients; areas of hyperalgesia which extended beyond the territory of the nerve also improved transiently (Marchettini et al, 1991). Carroll et al performed a non randomised cohort study on 71 patients with neuropathic pain with an objective to identify a subgroup of patients who are more responsive to IV lidocaine treatment by analysing differing pain qualities of neuropathic pain such as stabbing and heavy. Baseline heavy pain quality, but not stabbing quality predicted subsequent relief of pain intensity in response to lidocaine (Carroll, 2010). The predictive value of the lidocaine test for a positive oral trial of lidocaine congeners remains to be determined (Mao & Chen, 2000).

## 19. Side effects and limitations

The side effects are usually mild, dose-dependent, and always resolve with a decrease in the infusion rate or discontinuation of the drug. Tremor is a probably the first sign of toxicity. Other neurologic side effects include insomnia or drowsiness, light-headedness, dysarthria and slurred speech, ataxia, depression, agitation, change in sensorium, a change in personality, nystagmus, hallucinations, memory impairment, and emotional lability. Susceptibility increases in older adults or in those with heart failure, settings in which CNS levels are increased due to a reduced volume of distribution, and in patients with significant liver impairment in whom the metabolism of lidocaine is reduced. Seizures occur at a higher plasma level, but can occur at a lower concentration if lidocaine is given to patients receiving oral tocainide or mexiletine, which are congeners of lidocaine. Cardiac side effects are usually infrequent. The primary cardiovascular side effects include sinus slowing, asystole, hypotension, and shock. These problems are most often associated with overdosing or with the overly rapid administration of lidocaine. The elderly and those with significant pre-existing heart disease are at greatest risk.

There are several limitations and caveats with the use of IV lidocaine in chronic pain.

1. As a sodium channel blocker it is expected that it relieves pain which is mostly spontaneous in origin, but most studies show that is effects more on evoked pain.
2. There is known consistent results even when used with a similar condition on a different patient.
3. There seems to be a subgroup of patients who truly respond to IV lidocaine therapy. The challenge is to identify them.
4. Even in patients in whom it works, the duration of analgesia is short lasting (mostly hours).
5. This also needs resources to administer, monitor treatment.
6. Most of the orally available sodium channel blockers do not have the same results when used on patients responsive to lidocaine.

## 20. Conclusion

Lidocaine therapy is a promising therapy for patients with neuropathic pain. Its routine use cannot be still advised considering the evidence and limitations. However for a resistant and challenging neuropathic pain patient this option should be tried, at least to test the responsiveness and may be utilised on acute on chronic pain situations. Potentially it may also serve to identify true neuropathic pain responders from placebo responders.

## 21. Acknowledgement

I am thankful to Mr Michael Herman for assisting me in data collection and literature review.

## 22. References

Amr, YM. Multi-Day Low Dose Ketamine Infusion as Adjuvant to Oral Gabapentin in Spinal Cord Injury Related Chronic Pain: A Prospective, Randomized, Double Blind Trial, *Pain Physician,* 2010;13:245-49.

Attal N, Gaudé V, Brasseur L, Dupuy M, Guirimand F, Parker F, Bouhassira D. Intravenous lidocaine in central pain: a double-blind, placebo-controlled, psychophysical study. *Neurology.* 2000 Feb 8;54(3):564-74. .

Attal N, Rouaud J, Brasseur L, Chauvin M, Bouhassira D. Systemic lidocaine in pain due to peripheral nerve injury and predictors of response. *Neurology.* 2004 Jan 27;62(2):218-25.

Attal N, Rouaud J, Brasseur L, Chauvin M, Bouhassira D. Systemic lidocaine in pain due to peripheral nerve injury and predictors of response. *Neurology.* 2004 Jan 27;62(2):218-25.

Baad-Hansen, L., Juhl, GI., Jensen, TS., Brandsborg, B., & Svensson, P. Differential effect of intravenous S-ketamine and fentanyl on atypical odontalgia and capsaicin-evoked pain, *Pain,* 2007 May;129(1-2):46-54.

Backonja, M., Arndt, G., & Gombar, KA., et al. Response of chronic neuropathic pain syndromes to ketamine: a preliminary study, *Pain* 1994;56:51–7.

Baranowski AP, De Courcey J, Bonello E. A trial of intravenous lidocaine on the pain and allodynia of postherpetic neuralgia. *J Pain Symptom Manage.* 1999 Jun;17(6):429-33.

Bartlett EE, Hutaserani O. Xylocaine for the relief of postoperative pain. Anesth Analg 1961;40:296-304. Mao J, Chen LL. Systemic lidocaine for neuropathic pain relief. *Pain*. 2000 Jul;87(1):7-17.

Bell RF. Ketamine for chronic non-cancer pain. *Pain*. 2009 Feb;141(3):210-4.

Ben-Ari, A., Lewis, MC., & Davidson, E. Chronic Administration of Ketamine for Analgesia, *Journal of Pain and Palliative Care Pharmacotherapy,* Jan 2007, Vol. 21, No. 1: 7–14.

Bennett, GJ. (2000) Update on the neurophysiology of pain transmission and modulation: focus on the NMDA-receptor, *J Pain Symptom Manage,* 2000 Jan;19(1 Suppl):S2-6.

Blonk, MI., Koder, BG., Van den Bemt, PM., & Huygen, FJ. Use of oral ketamine in chronic pain management: a review, *Eur J Pain,* 2010 May;14(5):466-72.

Bruera E, Ripamonti C, Brenneis C, Macmillan K, Hanson J. A randomized double-blind crossover trial of intravenous lidocaine in the treatment of neuropathic cancer pain. *J Pain Symptom Manage*. 1992 Apr;7(3):138-40.

Carr, DB et al. Safety and efficacy of intranasal ketamine for the treatment of breakthrough pain in patients with chronic pain: a randomized, double-blind, placebo-controlled, crossover study. *Pain*. 2004 Mar;108(1-2):17-27

Carroll I. Intravenous lidocaine for neuropathic pain: diagnostic utility and therapeutic efficacy. *Curr Pain Headache Rep*. 2007 Feb;11(1):20-4.

Carroll IR, Younger JW, Mackey SC. Pain quality predicts lidocaine analgesia among patients with suspected neuropathic pain. *Pain Med*. 2010 Apr;11(4):617-21.

Castrillon, EE et al. Effect of peripheral NMDA receptor blockade with ketamine on chronic myofascial pain in temporomandibular disorder patients: a randomized, double-blinded, placebo-controlled trial. *J Orofac Pain*. 2008 Spring;22(2):122-30.

Chaplan SR, Bach FW, Shafer SL, Yaksh TL. Prolonged alleviation of tactile allodynia by intravenous lidocaine in neuropathic rats. *Anesthesiology* 1995;83:775-785.

Clements, JA., Nimmo, WS., & Grant, IS. Bioavailability, pharmacokinetics and analgesic activity of ketamine in humans, *J Pharm Sci,* 1982;71:539–42.

Cook, A.J., Woolf, C.J., Wall, P.D. & McMahon, S.B. Dynamic receptive field plasticity in rat spinal dorsal horn following C-primary afferent input, *Nature,* 325 (1987) 151–153.

Dahan et al. Population pharmacokinetic-pharmacodynamic modeling of ketamine-induced pain relief of chronic pain, *Eur J Pain,* 2011 Mar;15(3):258-67.

Devor M, Wall PD, Catalan N. Systemic lidocaine silences ectopic neuroma and DRG discharges without blocking nerve conduction. *Pain* 1992;48:261-268.

Devor M. Neuropathic pain and injured nerve: peripheral mechanisms. *Br Med Bull* 1991;47:619-630.

Dyck PJ. *Clinical features and differential diagnosis of peripheral neuropathy*. In: Dyck PJ, Thomas PK, Lambert EH, Bunge R, editors. Peripheral neuropathy, 2. Philadelphia, PA: W.B. Saunders, 1984. pp.1169-1190.

Ebert, B, Mikkelsen, S., Thorkildsen, C., & Borgbjerg, FM. Norketamine, the main metabolite of ketamine, is a non-competitive NMDA receptor antagonist in the rat cortex and spinal cord. *European J Pharmacology* 1997;333:99–104.

Eichenberger, U., Neff, F., & Sveticic, G., *et al*. Chronic phantom limb pain: The effects of calcitonin, ketamine, and their combination on pain and sensory thresholds. *Anesth Analg* 2008;106:1265–73.

Eide, PK., Jorum, E., Stubhaug, A., et al. Relief of post-herpetic neuralgia with the *N*-methyl-d-aspartic acid receptor antagonist ketamine: a double-blind, cross-over comparison with mor- phine and placebo, *Pain* 1994;58:347–54.

Eide, PK., Stubhaug, A., & Stenehjem, AE. Central dysesthesia pain after traumatic spinal cord injury is dependent on *N*-methyl-d- aspartate receptor activation. *Neurosurgery* 1995;37:1080–7.

Ellemann K, Sjögren P, Banning AM, Jensen TS, Smith T, Geertsen P. Trial of intravenous lidocaine on painful neuropathy in cancer patients. *Clin J Pain*. 1989 Dec;5(4):291-4.

Felsby, S., Nielsen, J., Arendt-Nielsen, L., & Jensen, TS. NMDA receptor blockade in chronic pain: a comparison of ketamine and magnesium chloride, *Pain* 1995;64:283–91.

Ferrante FM, Paggioli J, Cherukuri S, Arthur GR. The analgesic response to intravenous lidocaine in the treatment of neuropathic pain. *Anesth Analg*. 1996 Jan;82(1):91-7.

Finnerup NB, Biering-Sørensen F, Johannesen IL, Terkelsen AJ, Juhl GI, Kristensen AD, Sindrup SH, Bach FW, Jensen TS. Intravenous lidocaine relieves spinal cord injury pain: a randomized controlled trial. *Anesthesiology*. 2005 May;102(5):1023-30.

Fisher, K., Coderre, TJ., & Hagen, NA. Targeting the N-methyl-D-aspartate receptor for chronic pain management. Preclinical animal studies, recent clinical experience and future research directions. *J Pain Symptom Manage*. 2000 Nov;20(5):358-73.

Fitzgibbon EJ, Hall P, Schroder C, Seely J, Viola R. Low dose ketamine as an analgesic adjuvant in difficult pain syndromes: a strategy for conversion from parenteral to oral ketamine. *J Pain Symptom Manage*. 2002 Feb;23(2):165-70.

Furuhashi-Yonaha, A., Iida, H., Asano, T., Takeda, T., & Dohi, S. Short- and long-term efficacy of oral ketamine in eight chronic-pain patients, *Can J Anaesth*, 2002;49:886–7.

Galer BS, Harle J, Rowbotham MC. Response to intravenous lidocaine infusion predicts subsequent response to oral mexiletine: a prospective study. *J Pain Symptom Manage*. 1996 Sep;12(3):161-7.

Galer, Bradley S. MD; Miller, Kurt V. MD; Rowbotham, Michael C. MD. Response to intravenous lidocaine infusion differs based on clinical diagnosis and site of nervous system injury. *Neurology* 1993, 43:1233-1235.

Goldberg, ME., Torjman, MC., Schwartzman, RJ., Mager, DE., Wainer, IW. Pharmacodynamic profiles of ketamine (R)- and (S)- with 5-day inpatient infusion for the treatment of complex regional pain syndrome. *Pain Physician*. 2010 Jul-Aug;13(4):379-87.

Gormsen L, Finnerup NB, Almqvist PM, Jensen TS. The efficacy of the AMPA receptor antagonist NS1209 and lidocaine in nerve injury pain: a randomized, double-blind, placebo-controlled, three-way crossover study. *Anesth Analg*. 2009 Apr;108(4):1311-9.

Gottrup H, Bach FW, Juhl G, et al. Differential effect of ketamine and lidocaine on spontaneous and mechanical evoked pain in patients with nerve injury pain. *Anesthesiology* 2006;104:527–36.

Gottrup, H., Bach, FW., Juhl, G., *et al*. Differential effect of ketamine and lidocaine on spontaneous and mechanical evoked pain in patients with nerve injury pain, *Anesthesiology*, 2006;104:527–36.

Grant, IS., Nimmo, WS., & Clements,JA. Pharmacokinetics and analgesic effects of i.m. and oral ketamine. *Br.J. Anaesth.*, (1981), 53, 805.

Graven-Nielsen, T., Aspegren Kendall, S., Henriksson, KG., et al. Ketamine reduces muscle pain, temporal summation, and re- ferred pain in fibromyalgia patients, *Pain,* 2000;85:483–91.

Hocking, G., & Cousins, MJ. Ketamine in chronic pain management: an evidence-based review. *Anesth Analg*. 2003 Dec;97(6):1730-9.

Huge, V., Lauchart, M., Magerl, W., Schelling, G., Beyer, A., Thieme, D., & Azad, SC. Effects of low-dose intranasal (S)-ketamine in patients with neuropathic pain. *Eur J Pain.* 2010 Apr;14(4):387-94.

Jorum, E., Warncke, T., & Stubhaug, A. Cold allodynia and hyperalgesia in neuropathic pain: The effect of N-methyl-D-aspartate (NMDA) receptor antagonist ketamine—A double-blind, cross-over comparison with alfentanil and placebo, *Pain,* 2003;101:229–35.

Kastrup J, Petersen P, Dejgård A, Angelo HR, Hilsted J. Intravenous lidocaine infusion--a new treatment of chronic painful diabetic neuropathy? *Pain.* 1987 Jan;28(1):69-75.

Kate, JC., Anthony H. Dickenson. NMDA receptors and pain—Hopes for novel analgesics, *Regional Anesthesia and Pain Medicine,* Volume 24, Issue 6, November-December 1999

Kharasch, ED., & Labroo, R. Metabolism of ketamine stereoisomers by human liver microsomes. *Anesthesiology*. 1992;77:1201–7.

Klepstad P, Borchgrevink PC. Four years' treatment with ketamine and a trial of dextromethorphan in a patient with severe post-herpetic neuralgia. *Acta Anaesthesiol Scand*. 1997;41: 422- 6.

Kohrs, R., & Durieux, ME. Ketamine: teaching an old drug new tricks. *Anesth Analg*. 1998 Nov;87(5):1186-93

Kvarnström A, Karlsten R, Quiding H, Gordh T. The analgesic effect of intravenous ketamine and lidocaine on pain after spinal cord injury. *Acta Anaesthesiol Scand.* 2004 Apr;48(4):498-506.

Kvarnstrom A. Karlsten R. Quiding H. Emanuelsson BM. Gordh T. The effectiveness of intravenous ketamine and lidocaine on peripheral neuropathic pain. *Acta Anaesthesiol Scand*. 2003 Aug;47(7):868-77.

Kvarnström, A., Karlsten, R., Quiding, H., & Gordh, T. The analgesic effect of intravenous ketamine and lidocaine on pain after spinal cord injury, *Acta Anaesthesiol Scand,*. 2004 Apr;48(4):498-506.

Kvarnstrom, A., Karlsten, R., Quiding, H., Emanuelsson, BM., & Gordh, T. The effectiveness of intravenous ketamine and lidocaine on peripheral neuropathic pain, *Acta Anaesthesiol Scand,* 2003 Aug, 47(7):868-77.

Lemming, D., Sorensen, J., Graven-Nielsen, T., Lauber, R., Arendt-Nielsen, L., & Gerdle, B. Managing chronic whiplash associated pain with a combination of low-dose opioid (remifentanil) and NMDA-antagonist (ketamine), *Eur J Pain,* 2007 Oct, 11(7):719-32.

Lemming, D., Sorensen, J., Graven-Nielsen, T., Nielsen, LA., & Gerdle, B. The Responses to Pharmacological Challenges and Experimental Pain in Patients with Chronic Whiplash-Associated Pain, *The Clinical Journal of Pain,* 2005;21: 412-21.

Lemming, Dag, Jan Sorensen, Thomas Graven-Nielsen, Lars Arendt-Nielsen, and Bjorn Gerdle. The Responses to Pharmacological Challenges and Experimental Pain in Patients With Chronic Whiplash-Associated Pain. *Clin J Pain*. 2005;21: 412-21.

Leong MS, Solvason HB. Case report: limbic system activation by intravenous lidocaine in a patient with a complex regional pain syndrome and major depression. *Pain Med.* 2000 Dec;1(4):358-61.

Leung, A., Wallace, MS., Ridgeway, B., *et al.* Concentration-effect relationship of intravenous alfentanil and ketamine on peripheral neurosensory thresholds, allodynia and hyperalgesia of neuropathic pain, *Pain,* 2001;91:177–87.

Li, J., Simone, DA., & Larson, AA. Windup leads to characteristics of central sensitization, *Pain,* 1999 Jan;79(1):75-82

Mao J, Chen LL. Systemic lidocaine for neuropathic pain relief. *Pain.* 2000 Jul;87(1):7-17.

Marchettini P, Lacerenza M, Marangoni C, Pellegata G, Sotgiu ML, Smirne S. Lidocaine test in neuralgia. *Pain.* 1992 Mar;48(3):377-82.

Max, MB., Byas-Smith, M., Gracely, RH., & Bennett, GJ. Intravenous infusion of the NMDA antagonist, ketamine, in chronic post- traumatic pain with allodynia; a double-blind comparison to alfentanil and placebo, *Clin Neuropharmacol,* 1995;18:360–8.

Medrik-Goldberg T, Lifschitz D, Pud D, Adler R, Eisenberg E. Intravenous lidocaine, amantadine, and placebo in the treatment of sciatica: a double-blind, randomized, controlled study. *Reg Anesth Pain Med.* 1999 Nov-Dec;24(6):534- 40.

Mercadante, S., Arcuri, E., Tirelli, W., & Casuccio, A. Analgesic effect of intravenous ketamine in cancer patients on morphine therapy: a randomized, controlled, double-blind, crossover, double-dose study. *J Pain Symptom Manage.* 2000 Oct;20(4):246-52.

Mercadante, S., Arcuri, E., Tirelli, W., & Casuccio, A. Analgesic effect of intravenous ketamine in cancer patients on morphine therapy: a randomized, controlled, double-blind, crossover, double-dose study, *J Pain Symptom Manage,* 2000 Oct, 20(4):246-52.

Mitchell, AC., & Fallon, MT. A single infusion of intravenous ketamine improves pain relief in patients with critical limb ischaemia: results of a double blind randomised controlled trial. *Pain.* 2002 Jun;97(3):275-81.

Nicolodi, M, & Sicuteri, F. Exploration of NMDA receptors in migraine: therapeutic and theoretic implications. *Int J Clin Pharmacol Res.* 1995;15(5-6):181-9.

Nikolajsen, L., Hansen, CL., Nielsen, J., Keller, J., Arendt-Nielsen, L., & Jensen, TS. The effect of ketamine on phantom pain: a central neuropathic disorder maintained by peripheral input. *Pain* 1996;67:69–77.

Nordin M, Nystrom B, Wallin U, Hagbarth KE. Ectopic sensory discharges and paresthesia in patients with disorders of peripheral nerves, dorsal roots and dorsal column. *Pain* 1984;20:231-245.

Oga, K., Kojima, T., Matsuura, M., Nagashima, M., Kato, J., Saeki, S., & Ogawa, S. Effects of low-dose ketamine on neuropathic pain: An electroencephalogram-electrooculogram/behavioral study, *Psychiatry Clin Neurosci,* 2002 Aug;56(4):355-63.

Okon, T. Ketamine: an introduction for the pain and palliative medicine physician, *Pain Physician.* 2007 May;10(3):493-500.

Orser, BA., Pennefather, PS. & MacDonald JF. (1997 Apr). Multiple mechanisms of ketamine blockade of N-methyl-D-aspartate receptors, *Anesthesiology,* 86(4), 903-17.

Persson,J., Hasselstrom, J., & Wiklund, B., et al. The analgesic effect of racemic ketamine in patients with chronic ischaemic pain due to lower extremity arteriosclerosis obliterans. *Acta Anaesthesiol Scand* 1998;42:750–8

Petrenko, AB., Yamakura, T., Baba, H., Shimoji, K. The role of N-methyl-D-aspartate (NMDA) receptors in pain: a review, *Anesth Analg*, 2003 Oct;97(4):1108-16.

Rathmell JP, Ballantyne JC. Local anesthetics for the treatment of neuropathic pain: on the limits of meta-analysis. *Anesth Analg*. 2005 Dec;101(6):1736-7.

Rowbotham MC, Reisner-Keller LA, Fields HL. Both intravenous lidocaine and morphine reduce the pain of postherpetic neuralgia. *Neurology*. 1991 Jul;41(7):1024-8.

Sabia, M., Hirsh, RA., Torjman, MC., Wainer, IW., Cooper, N., Domsky, R., & Goldberg, ME.,. Advances in translational neuropathic research: example of enantioselective pharmacokinetic-pharmacodynamic modeling of ketamine-induced pain relief in complex regional pain syndrome, *Curr Pain Headache Rep*, 2011 Jun;15(3):207-14.

Schnider T, Gaeta TW, Brose RR, et al.: Derivation and cross-validation of pharmacokinetic parameters for computer- controlled infusion of lidocaine in pain therapy. *Anesthesiology* 1996, 84:1043–1050.

Scholz A. Mechanisms of (local) anaesthetics on voltage-gated sodium and other ion channels. *Br J Anaesth*. 2002 Jul;89(1):52- 61.

Schwartzman, RJ., Alexander, GM., Grothusen, JR., *et al*. Outpatient intravenous ketamine for the treatment of complex regional pain syndrome: A double-blind placebo controlled study, *Pain*, 2009;147:107–15.

Scrivani SJ, Chaudry A, Maciewicz RJ, Keith DA. Chronic neurogenic facial pain: lack of response to intravenous phentolamine. *J Orofac Pain*. 1999 Spring;13(2):89-96.

Sharma S, Rajagopal MR, Palat G, Singh C, Haji AG, Jain D. A phase II pilot study to evaluate use of intravenous lidocaine for opioid-refractory pain in cancer patients. *J Pain Symptom Manage*. 2009 Jan;37(1):85-93.

Sigtermans, MJ., Van Hilten, JJ., Bauer, MC., Arbous, MS., Marinus, J., Sarton, EY., & Dahan, A. Ketamine produces effective and long-term pain relief in patients with Complex Regional Pain Syndrome Type 1, *Pain*, 2009 Oct;145(3):304-11.

Sinner, B., Graf, BM., Schuttler, J. & Schwilden, H. (2008). Ketamine in Modern anesthetics, *Handbook of experimental pharmacology*, vol 182. Springer-Verlag. Berlin Heidelberg, pp 313-333.

Sinnott CJ, Gar®eld JM, Strichartz GR. Differential efficacy of intravenous lidocaine in alleviating ipsilateral versus contralateral neuropathic pain in the rat. *Pain* 1999;80:521-531.

Sörensen, J., Bengtsson, A., Ahlner, J., Henriksson, KG., Ekselius, L., & Bengtsson M. Fibromyalgia--are there different mechanisms in the processing of pain? A double blind crossover comparison of analgesic drugs, *J Rheumatol*, 1997 Aug;24(8):1615-21.

Soto E, et al. [Epub ahead of print] Oral Ketamine in the Palliative Care Setting: A Review of the Literature and Case Report of a Patient With Neurofibromatosis Type 1 and Glomus Tumor-Associated Complex Regional Pain Syndrome, *Am J Hosp Palliat Care*, 2011 Jul 29.

Tremont-Lukats IW, Challapalli V, McNicol ED, Lau J, Carr DB. Systemic administration of local anesthetics to relieve neuropathic pain: a systematic review and meta-analysis. *Anesth Analg.* 2005 Dec;101(6):1738-49.

Tremont-Lukats IW, Hutson PR, Backonja MM. A randomized, double-masked, placebo-controlled pilot trial of extended IV lidocaine infusion for relief of ongoing neuropathic pain. *Clin J Pain.* 2006 Mar-Apr;22(3):266-71.

Tverskoy M, Oren M, Vaskovich M, et al. Ketamine enhances local anesthetic and analgesic effects of bupivacaine by peripheral mechanism: a study in postoperative patients. Neurosci Lett 1996;215:5–8.

Ushida, T., Tani, T., & Kanbara T, et al. Analgesic effects of ketamine ointment in patients with complex regional pain syndrome type 1. *Reg Anesth Pain Med* 2002;27:524–8.

Viola V, Newnham HH, Simpson RW. Treatment of intractable painful diabetic neuropathy with intravenous lignocaine. *J Diabetes Complications.* 2006 Jan-Feb;20(1):34-9.

Wall PD, Gutnick M. Properties of afferent nerve impulses originating from a neuroma. *Nature* 1974;248:740-743. Devor M. Neuropathic pain and injured nerve: peripheral mechanisms. *Br Med Bull* 1991;47:619-630.

Wallace MS, Dyck JB, Rossi SS, Yaksh TL. Computer-controlled lidocaine infusion for the evaluation of neuropathic pain after peripheral nerve injury. *Pain.* 1996 Jul;66(1):69-77.

Wallace MS, Ridgeway BM, Leung AY, Gerayli A, Yaksh TL. Concentration-effect relationship of intravenous lidocaine on the allodynia of complex regional pain syndrome types I and II. *Anesthesiology.* 2000 Jan;92(1):75-83.

Warncke, T., Jorum, E., & Stubhaug, A. Local treatment with the *N*-methyl-d-aspartate receptor antagonist ketamine, inhibit development of secondary hyperalgesia in man by a peripheral action. *Neurosci Lett* 1997;227:1–4.

White, PF. Ketamine: its pharmacology and therapeutic uses. *Anesthesiology* 1982;56:119-36.

White, PF., Schuttler, J. & Shafer, A., et al. Comparative pharmacology of the ketamine isomers: studies in volunteers, *Br J Anaesth,* 1985;57:197-203.

Wood JN, Boorman JP, Okuse K, Baker MD.Voltage-gated sodium channels and pain pathways. *J Neurobiol.* 2004 Oct;61(1):55-71.

Woolf CJ, Wiesenfeld-Hallin Z. The systemic administration of local anesthetics produces a selective depression of C-afferent fiber evoked activity in the spinal cord. Pain *1985;*23:361-374.

Wu CL, Tella P, Staats PS, Vaslav R, Kazim DA, Wesselmann U, Raja SN. Analgesic effects of intravenous lidocaine and morphine on postamputation pain: a randomized double-blind, active placebo-controlled, crossover trial. *Anesthesiology.* 2002 Apr;96(4):841-8.

Yamamoto, T., Katayama, Y., Hirayama, T., & Tsubokawa, T. Pharmacological classification of central post-stroke pain: comparison with the results of chronic motor cortex stimulation therapy, *Pain,* 1997 Aug;72(1-2):5-12.

Yanagihara, Y., Ohtani, M., Kariya, S., Uchino, K., & Hiraishi T, et al. Plasma concentration profiles of ketamine and norketamine after administration of various ketamine preparations to healthy Japanese volunteers. *Biopharm Drug Dispos.* 2003;24:37–43.

Zhou, HY., Chen, SR., & Pan, HL. Targeting N-methyl-D-aspartate receptors for treatment of neuropathic pain, *Expert Rev Clin Pharmaco,* 2011 May 1;4(3):379-388.

Zhou, S., Bonasera, L., & Carlton, SM. Peripheral administration of NMDA, AMPA or KA results in pain behaviors in rats. *Neuroreport* 1996;7:895–900.

# 4

# Cannabinoids and Neuropathic Pain

P.W. Brownjohn and J.C. Ashton
*Department of Pharmacology & Toxicology, University of Otago*
*New Zealand*

## 1. Introduction

Cannabinoids are drugs that are either derived from cannabis or that induce similar behavioural and physiological effects to cannabis. They fall into three classes: those that are produced by plants of the *Cannabis* genus, termed phytocannabinoids (plant cannabinoids); those that are produced within the body, termed endocannabinoids (endogenous cannabinoids); and those that are produced synthetically to mimic the pharmacology of naturally occurring cannabinoids.

Cannabinoids stand in relation to cannabis as opioids such as codeine, pethidine, fentanyl, and methadone stand in relation to opium. While opium and opioids are used and abused recreationally, opioids have long been at the forefront of first line analgesia for acute and chronic pain indications. Similarly, while cannabis and synthetic analogues are drugs of abuse, cannabinoids also have beneficial therapeutic effects. While the therapeutic effects of cannabinoids do not yet approach those of opioids, there has been extensive pharmaceutical research into the use of cannabinoids for the treatment of pain. In contrast with opioids, however, there is mounting evidence that cannabinoids may be more efficacious in the treatment of chronic pain conditions, such as neuropathies, rather than acute pain.

## 2. Cannabinoid pharmacology

### 2.1 A brief history

Phytocannabinoids are derived from the *Cannabis* species, primarily *Cannabis sativa* which originated in China and Central and South Asia. Two other species are known; *C. indica* and *C. Ruderalis*, and possibly a third; *C. afghanica*. Of these, *C. sativa* is the largest and most diverse genus (Clarke *et al.*, 2002). Cannabis was probably first used as a medicinal herb in India around 800BC, and in Persia and Tibet by 500BC, purportedly as an anaesthetic during surgery, while the therapeutic properties of cannabis were first recorded in China as early as 200 AD. It wasn't until the nineteenth century, however, that the Irish doctor William O'Shaughnessy began the scientific investigation of the chemical properties of cannabis (Frankhauser, 2002).

By 1900 various pharmaceutical companies in Europe were promoting cannabis based products for the treatment of migraine, menstrual cramps, whooping cough, asthma, and as a sedative and soporific. During the twentieth century, however, cannabis lost favor as a medicine due to combination of the development of better drugs, the instability of cannabis drug formulations, unfavorable economics, and legal restrictions on its availability (Frankhauser, 2002). Today, cannabis and cannabinoids are once again the subject of serious pharmaceutical development. More targeted drug formulations, a greater understanding of the evidence base for cannabinoid efficacy and safety for particular conditions, and the development of wholly new ways of manipulating the endocannabinoid system have lead to a resurgence of research.

Following the initiation of the scientific study of cannabinoid chemistry in 1838 by O'Shaughnessy (Di Marzo, 2006a), the first purified cannabinoid, named cannabinol, was isolated in 1899, and by 1932, its structure had been partially described. In 1964 Raphael Mechoulam, at Hebrew University in Israel, described the structure of the principle pharmacologically active component of cannabis, delta-9-tetrahydrocannabinol (THC) (Mechoulam *et al.*, 1965). Following this critical discovery, the study of the pharmacological effects of cannabis and cannabinoids accelerated from 1970 through to the 1990s. This period of cannabinoid pharmacology clarified the behavioural and physiological effects of cannabis and classical cannabinoids, in particular THC.

It had already been discovered that opium derived opioids interact with an endogenous receptor system, mimicking the actions of endogenous opioids. It was hypothesised that a similar receptor binding system might underlie the effects of cannabinoids, and in 1988, Devane and colleagues (Devane et al., 1988) published an article describing and characterising binding sites for THC. This rapidly led to the discovery of a specific cannabinoid receptor, subsequently termed cannabinoid receptor I, or CB1, in 1990 (Herkenham *et al.*, 1990a). A seminal study by Herkenham and colleagues (Herkenham *et al.*, 1990a) used autoradiographical binding to describe the distribution of CB1 receptors throughout the rat brain. Soon afterward, a similar distribution of CB1 receptors was described for the human brain by Glass and colleagues (Glass et al., 1997). The results of these studies helped explain many of the psychoactive effects of cannabinoids that had been previously characterized.

The discovery of the CB1 receptor gave impetus to the search for endogenous cannabinoids for which CB1 would be the natural target. The first endogenous ligand discovered and characterised for this receptor was a lipid, arachidonoylethanolamide, discovered in 1992, and given the name anandamide after the Sanskrit word for bliss, *ananda* (Devane et al., 1992). Anandamide is not stored in vesicles like classical neurotransmitters, and is instead synthesized in neurons on demand primarily via a two step reaction, catalysed by N-acyltransferase and a member of the phospholipase D family, N-acylphosphatidylethanolamine (Okamoto et al., 2007). It is a highly lipophilic derivative of arachidonic acid and readily diffuses across the plasma membrane upon synthesis, activating CB1 receptors before rapid enzymatic hydrolysis by fatty acid amide hydrolase (FAAH) (Cravatt et al., 1996). This makes anandamide ideally adapted for signaling pathways that require a rapid and local response, such as the regulation of neuronal excitability in the brain, or the modulation of vascular tone. A second endocannabinoid, 2-arachodonalglycerol (2-AG), was discovered in 1995 (Mechoulam et al., 1995). Like anandamide, synthesis and degradation of 2-AG is enzymatically regulated, in this instance primarily by diacylglycerol lipase α and β, and monoglyceride lipase (Dinh et al., 2002), respectively. More recently there have been at least four additional endocannabinoids suggested: 2-arachidonyl-glycerolether (noladin, 2-AGE), *O*-arachidonyl-ethanolamine (virohdamine), *N*-arachidonoyl-dopamine (NADA) (Pacher et al., 2006), and the sleep inducing oleic acid derivative oleamide (Lees *et al.*, 2004), although these have not been as extensively characterized as anandamide and 2-AG.

A second cannabinoid receptor, cannabinoid receptor II (CB2), was discovered in 1992 (Munro et al., 1993). Unlike CB1, CB2 appeared to be abundant in immune cells of the spleen (lymphocytes) and tonsils but not in the brain (Galiegue, 1995). This finding helped explain another of the pharmacological effects of cannabis; suppression of the immune system.

### 2.2 Cannabinoid receptors

CB1 occurs in deuterostome invertebrate animals as well as in vertebrates, which suggests that the endocannabinoid system developed early in evolutionary history and is therefore likely to be fundamental to a variety of basic physiological processes (Elphick *et al.*, 2001). These include processes that are mainly involved with both the central and peripheral nervous systems, though CB1 is most densely expressed in the central nervous system (CNS). In addition to the psychoactive effects of CB1 activation in the brain, CB1 receptors have a number of functions in other organ systems. CB1 is co-expressed with CB2 in many immune cells, including monocytes and microglia. Some researchers have suggested that CB1 may be constitutively expressed in immune cells, and respond to initial injury signals, and that a second receptor, CB2, is induced during inflammation or immune functions (Cabral *et al.*, 2005). CB1 receptors are in fact expressed in a great many tissues throughout the body, including in the eye (where they help regulate intraocular pressure), the placenta, gonads and reproductive system, skin, and in nerves terminating in the gut wall (Izzo *et al.*, 2001; Park *et al.*, 2003; Njie *et al.*, 2006). There are also CB1 receptors in cardiac muscle, blood vessels, and on peripheral nerves of the cardiovascular system.

CB2 was characterized shortly after CB1 (Munro et al., 1993). CB2 receptors are found at the highest densities in immune cells, and as such, spleen and tonsil homogenates show very high levels of CB2 protein. For this reason, CB2 has come to be referred to as the cannabinoid immune receptor, contrasting with CB1 as the cannabinoid central nervous system receptor. There are exceptions to this however: as noted CB1 is found in a variety of tissues including immune cells, and CB2 has been found to be important in the proliferation and differentiation of immature neurons. Because CB2 is located for the most part in peripheral tissues and in immune cells in particular, CB2 represents an attractive target for the immunomodulatory and anti-inflammatory effects of cannabinoids, but without the psychoactive effects caused by CB1 activation.

Although CB2 expression is well characterized in the immune system (Galiegue et al., 1995), the expression of the CB2 receptor in the brain is still an area of controversy. It is known now that CB2 are definitely expressed in microglia, which are resident immune cells in the CNS (Cabral *et al.*, 2005). CB2 has been detected in microglia in neuritic plaques in brains taken from patients that have died with Alzheimer's disease (Benito et al., 2003). More controversially, CB2 receptors have also been reported on neurons of rodents and mustelids (Van Sickle *et al.*, 2005; Gong *et al.*, 2006; Onaivi *et al.*, 2006).

CB1 and CB2 are G protein coupled receptors (GPCRs), linked to inhibitory Gi proteins. Activation of these receptors inhibits the accumulation of the messenger molecule cyclic adenosine monophosphate (cAMP) in cells, via inhibition of adenylyl cyclase (Scotter et al.,

2006). GPCRs are extremely abundant and variable, but share the same basic structure; which is an extracellular N terminus, an intracellular C terminus, seven hydrophobic trans-plasma membrane helical domains, three extracellular loops, and three intracellular loops. Cellular signalling pathways for CB1 are well studied; less so for CB2. Stimulation of the CB1 receptor inhibits the influx of $Ca^{2+}$ into cells by way of a variety of voltage sensitive $Ca^{2+}$ channels (VSCCs). In the brain, depolarization of postsynaptic neurons can cause a release of endocannabinoids that act as reverse neurotransmitters to presynaptic CB1 receptors, reducing neurotransmitter release from presynaptic neurons. As CB1 receptors are present on both excitatory and inhibitory neurons, its activation can have diverse and often opposing effects in the central nervous system. CB1 is also coupled to G protein-coupled inwardly rectifying potassium channels (GIRKs), and this tends to hyperpolarize presynaptic neuron terminals, and contributes to the reduction in excitation/inhibition of post-synaptic neurons. Inhibition of VSCCs has also been implicated as a key mechanism by which vascular CB1 receptors mediate vasodilation.

It is important to remember that much of the research that has been done on cannabinoid receptors has been done on those found in rodents, particularly rats. The amino acid sequence for CB1 is very similar in rats and humans, with 97% sequence identity between the two species (Gerard et al., 1991). Although CB1 is highly conserved between species, the same cannot be said for CB2. CB2 has diverged a great deal more between species than CB1, with only 81% sequence identity between the rat and human receptors (Griffin et al., 2000). Modeling the receptors has shown that there is some 87% identity between the rat and human receptors in the transmembrane regions, which are critical for drug binding. Therefore, although CB1 rat models are often (but not always) good predictors of how a drug will perform for human CB1 receptors, this is not so frequently the case for CB2. Drugs that show promising selectivity for CB2 that have only been tested in rodents should therefore be treated with caution when extrapolating possible effects in humans.

While CB1 and CB2 are two undisputed and well characterised members of the cannabinoid receptor family by which cannabinoids exert their effects, there is evidence of cannabinoid binding to additional targets. Some effects by cannabinoids in experiments do not appear to be mediated by either CB1 or CB2. In particular, the endocannabinoid anandamide may act on a variety of targets including a number of orphaned GPCRs (such GPR55, GPR112) T-type $Ca^{2+}$ channels, $Na^{2+}$ channels, Transient Receptor Potential Vanilloid type 1 (TRPV1) channels, $\alpha$7-nicotinic acetylcholine receptors, and background and voltage-gated $K^+$ channels (van der Stelt *et al.*, 2005).

Although cannabinoid analgesia has been reasonably well studied in humans (Pertwee, 2001; Burns *et al.*, 2006; Huskey, 2006; Manzanares *et al.*, 2006) the exact contributions of the cannabinoid receptors is still under investigation. Many preclinical studies have shown that cannabinoids produce analgesia by acting in both the central and peripheral nervous system (Pertwee, 2001), via CB1 receptors in the brain, but also by both CB1 and CB2 receptors in the spinal cord and periphery (Agarwal et al., 2007).

### 2.3 Cannabinoids

Cannabinoids tend to fall into five major structural classes: The classical cannabinoids (including phytocannabinoids), bicyclic and tricyclic analogues, endocannabinoids, aminoalkylindoles, and diarylpyrazoles. While classical cannabinoids are based on the structure of phytocannabinoids, the other four classes of ligand are not, and tend to have a non-classical structure.

The first classical cannabinoids were the phytocannabinoids purified from the cannabis plant, *C.sativa*. At least 483 different natural chemicals have been extracted and purifed from cannabis and of these, phytocannabinoids are exclusively found in cannabis plants. At the time of writing, 66 distinct phytocannabinoids have been isolated and purified from *C.sativa*. These include THC and cannabidiol, which have been extensively studied for their medicinal qualities. Dronabinol is the name given to the synthetically produced (-)-*trans*-isomer of THC (which is also naturally occurring), while nabilone, also a classical cannabinoid, is a synthetically produced potent analogue of THC. Both dronabinol and nabilone are currently licensed medications, and are discussed later.

With the characterisation of specific cannabinoid receptors, it was possible to develop synthetic compounds tailored directly to the cannabinoid receptors, which differed from the classical cannabinoid structure. Bicyclic and tricyclic synthetic cannabinoids of the non-classical type make up the second group of cannabinoid ligands. Chief among agonists of this group, CP55,940 was developed by Pfizer in 1974, and is a bicyclic cannabinoid, without the middle dihydropyran ring of the classical tricyclic cannabinoids. These were altered further by the substitution of additional hydroxyl groups for added capability to form hydrogen bonds. CP55,940 is considerably more potent as an agonist at both cannabinoid receptors compared with THC. As a result, the psychoactive effects of CP55,940 are far more intense than those caused by THC (which is a relatively weak cannabinoid receptor agonist) and therefore CP55,940 has not been suitable for clinical use. Unlike dronabinol and nabilone, CP55,940 and other drugs like it have never been marketed because they are extremely psychoactive (i.e., cause profound effects on the central nervous system).

Levonantradol is a tricyclic cannabinoid that was produced by Pfizer, and differs from THC not only in that it has additional hydrogen binding sites, but also in that it has an aromatic group attached to the alkyl tail. Levonantradol is considerably more potent than THC, and unlike CP55,940, was used in clinical tests. Levonantradol was found to provide considerable pain relief for patients after operations, but had more intense side effects than THC (Jain et al., 1981). Another potent tricyclic THC analogue that has been used extensively in studying the endocannabinoid system is HU-210. With a long duration of action, and exhibiting 100-800 times more potency than THC, it is unsuitable for human use. Like other potent synthetic cannabinoids HU-210 has a high degree of oxygen substitution compared with phytocannabinoids. Ajulemic acid is compound that is related to HU-210, and is a synthetic derivative of the active metabolite of THC, 11-carboxy-THC. Ajulemic acid is similar in structure to HU-210, but has a carboxylate substituted for the methyl hydroxyl substituent at position 9. Ajulemic acid has been administered to humans in clinical tests, and has been found to have promise for the control of neuropathic pain.

Synthetic cannabinoids were initially developed based on the classical cannabinoid structural template (Di Marzo, 2006b). Phytocannabinoids are highly lipophilic and show extremely high levels of non-specific binding in radio-ligand binding experiments. Highly potent synthetic analogues of THC are often more polar than phytocannabinoids, and able to form more hydrogen bonds. Because THC and its derivatives tend to be highly lipophilic, it accumulates in cell membranes when it is applied to sectioned or homogenised tissues. For many years, this made it difficult to identify and characterise the specific binding sites for cannabinoids, which hindered study of the endocannabinoid system. Identification of cannabinoid receptors and their distribution in the body has been greatly facilitated by the discovery of high affinity compounds such as CP 55,940. Radio-labeled CP 55,940 was the compound used by Devane and colleagues (Devane et al., 1988) in the breakthrough work that lead to the characterisation CB1, and by Herkenham and colleagues to describe the distribution of CB1 in the rat brain (Herkenham *et al.*, 1990b).

A third group of cannabinoids consists of endocannabinoids, which were first identified soon after the characterisation of cannabinoid receptors (Di Marzo, 2006b). The prototypical endocannabinoid is anandamide and has been extensively studied for both its biochemistry and pharmacology. Anandamide consists of a long hydrophobic alkyl tail, and an ethanolamide head group. The endocannabinoid 2-AG differs from anandamide by the addition of a second hydroxyl at the headgroup, and an ester group replacing the amide. Anandamide appears to have several-fold greater potency than 2-AG, though there is enormous variation in published results.

A fourth category of cannabinoids, bearing little structural similarity to either classical cannabinoids or endocannabinoids are aminoalkylindoles, the most commonly used of which is WIN55,212-2, which is a potent agonist at both CB1 and CB2 receptors, but shows some degree of selectivity for CB2. JWH-133 is another potent indole that is part of a family of compounds named after their discoverer, JW Huffman, and shows a high degree of selectivity (200-fold) for CB2 (Huffman, 2005).

Non-classical ligand development also included, for the first time, receptor subtype selective antagonists. Developed by Sanofi-Recherche in the 1990s, SR141716A (later SR141716) and SR144528 are highly selective antagonists against CB1 and CB2, respectively, and are members of the fifth main category of cannabinoids, the diarylpyrazoles (Rinaldi-Carmona et al., 1994). By virtue of selectively excluding the actions of one of the cannabinoid receptors, these two compounds have been instrumental in critical research that has furthered our understanding of cannabinoid pharmacology. Indeed these agonists were used to provide definitive evidence that CP 55,940 causes its effects through the same biochemical pathways as THC, in experiments that show that its psychoactive effects are completely blocked by the CB1 receptor antagonist SR141716 (Compton et al., 1992).

Knowledge of receptor selectivity is important for the medicinal use of cannabinoids because CB1 and CB2 have distinct distributions and distinct physiological effects; CB1 is chiefly responsible for the psychoactive effects of cannabinoids and CB2 is mainly involved in the anti-inflammatory and immunomodulatory effects of cannabinoids. Development of subtype selective ligands will be discussed in a later chapter.

## 3. Cannabis and cannabinoids in the clinic

### 3.1 Cannabis

Most of the higher quality evidence for the antinociceptive effects of cannabinoids in humans comes from studies using licensed cannabinoid drugs, rather than with medical cannabis. Very few clinical trial data for smoked cannabis exist, though there are some for

HIV-induced neuropathy (Abrams et al., 2007) and experimental pain (Hill *et al.*, 1974; Wallace *et al.*, 2007). It is also difficult to interpret case histories and patient or doctor testimonies, mostly because of the lack of placebo controls, but also because habitual cannabis users can develop tolerance to many of the effects of the drug. Moreover, the amount of active cannabinoids in any given cannabis cigarette is highly variable: THC content in raw cannabis often ranges between 1.5 and 3.7%; the size of the cannabis cigarettes can vary; and the amount of cigarette smoked at any one time can vary.

### 3.2 Licensed formulations

The cannabinoid drugs that were first approved for clinical use were synthetic analogues or stereoisomers of THC. These are the (-)-*trans*-isomer of THC, dronabinol (Marinol™, Namisol®), and the more potent THC analogue, nabilone (Cesamet™). Both dronabinol and nabilone are used clinically in several countries, especially in palliative care. This abstracts from the ability of cannabis to reduce nausea and vomiting after treatment with anti-cancer medicines (Machado Rocha et al., 2008). There is good evidence and justification for the continued use of cannabinoids in the treatment of nausea and vomiting in patients receiving chemotherapy, especially in those patients whose nausea and emesis does not respond to other treatments. In addition to anti-emetic action, they are also used as appetite stimulants in wasting conditions such as HIV/AIDS. Another THC analogue, levonantradol, has both anti-emetic and powerful analgesic properties. It was effective in the treatment of post surgical pain (Jain et al., 1981), and as an antiemetic in cancer patients (Cronin *et al.*, 1981; Hutcheon *et al.*, 1983; Stambaugh *et al.*, 1984). However, adverse events were common, and sometimes severe and dose limiting (Cronin *et al.*, 1981; Hutcheon *et al.*, 1983), thus the drug was judged unacceptable and the programme was dropped (Dr K. Koe quoted in (Iversen, 2000)).

Marinol is an oral form of dronabinol that is manufactured by Unimed Pharmaceuticals, and is available in the United States, Canada, and in some European countries. Marinol comes as capsules with the dronabinol dissolved in sesame seed oil. These are available in sizes of 2.5, 5 and 10 mg. In an effort to improve the pharmacokinetic profile of orally administered dronabinol, Echo Pharmaceuticals in The Netherlands has developed Namisol, a preparation of dronabinol formulated with an emulsifier in oral tablets. The company is currently preparing phase II clinical trials of Namisol in neuropathic pain, multiple sclerosis and Alzheimer's disease. Nabilone is marketed under the name Cesamet, which is a registered trademark of Valeant Pharmaceuticals International. Cesamet comes in the form of crystalline powder capsules, containing 1 mg nabilone, and is available in the UK, Canada, and in some European countries.

A unique cannabinoid preparation that is currently in clinical use is GW Pharmaceutical's cannabis-plant derived medicine, Sativex™ (GW-1000). This is a natural preparation that standardises THC with cannabidiol in a fixed ratio (1:1.08) and is administered using sublingual sprays or tablets, and oromucosal or oropharyngeal sprays (Smith, 2004). Cannabidiol is thought to have a quite different mechanism of action to THC, and so Sativex is a more complex drug than the pure form of THC or THC analogues. In theory, cannabidiol should work in synergy with THC to increase some of its beneficial effects, and reduce some of its adverse effects. By using a whole plant extract, GW Pharmaceuticals hope to retain some of the putative properties of whole cannabis, as opposed to isolated THC, but in concentrations that are below that which are thought to cause the major detrimental effects of cannabis. By combining THC and cannabidiol in a fixed ratio, and processing the whole plant extract such that concentrations are precisely specified, Sativex can be administered as a metered and recordable dose, unlike cannabis. Sativex has been approved for use in Canada as a treatment to help reduce pain and tremor in patients with multiple sclerosis, and has been approved for off label use in other countries. Similarly, Cannador® consists of capsules containing a standardized cannabis extract, with a 2:1 ratio of THC to cannabidiol. The cannabis has been grown in Switzerland and processed in Germany, organised by the Institute for Clinical Research (IKF) in Berlin. While Cannador has been used in clinical testing for a number of indications, it has not been licensed for therapeutic use.

While many cannabinoid formulations are not specifically licensed for pain conditions, managing pain is a very useful side effect of cannabinoids used in palliative care in conditions such as HIV/AIDS and multiple sclerosis, and for the adverse effects of chemotherapy. HIV infection is a well known cause of periperheral neuropathies, while multiple sclerosis is a demyelinating neurodegenerative disorder that can also cause serious neuropathic path. Some chemotherapeutics can also cause neuropathies and chronic pain, for example paclitaxel (taxol), a frontline anticancer therapeutic.

### 3.3 Pharmacokinetics

When smoked, 10 to 25% of the THC content of cannabis leaf is absorbed into the bloodstream (Adams *et al.*, 1996). Via the inhalation route, THC reaches peak levels much faster, and ultimately reaches higher peak plasma concentrations than via oral or even oromucosal administration of THC. In one study, smoking cannabis resulted in peak plasma concentrations of THC more than 10 times greater than an equivalent dose of THC given by oromucosal spray, and peak plasma concentrations were reached within 9 minutes, compared to 180 minutes (Robson, 2005). The high peak plasma concentrations of THC that are achieved very rapidly by smoking cannabis may help explain why some users claim that the medical benefits of smoked cannabis are greater than for other THC preparations (Medicines and Healthcare products Regulatory Agency, 2007). However, the "peak and trough" pharmacokinetics of smoked cannabis means that users experience significantly greater psychoactivity than when using Sativex, where gradual dose titration to steady state plasma concentrations is possible.

Via the oral route, cannabinoids are absorbed much more slowly than via the inhalation route, yet tend to have a longer duration of action. Nabilone and dronabinol are both highly lipophilic compounds, with similar pharmacokinetic profiles when delivered orally. While nabilone and dronabinol have a similar time to onset of action (60 – 90 min and 30 – 60 min, respectively) and peak plasma concentration (2 hours and 2 - 4 hours, respectively), nabilone has a longer duration of action (8 - 12 hours versus 4 – 6 hours, respectively), allowing less frequent dosing. A typical dosing regimen for nabilone in the treatment of chemotherapy-induced nausea and vomiting is 1-2 mg taken 1 to 3 hours prior to chemotherapy and 2 times a day for up to 2 days afterward. For dronabinol, 5 mg may be given 1 to 3 hours before chemotherapy, and every 2 to 4 hours afterwards for a total of 4 to 6 doses each day.

Because cannabinoids are highly lipophilic and pass easily through biological membranes, they can be administered using sublingual sprays or tablets, and oropharyngeal or oromucosal sprays, as Sativex is. This avoids both first pass metabolism that occurs in oral administration, and the problems associated with smoking and pulmonary administration, while retaining rapid uptake into the blood stream and dispersal around the body and the nervous system that is characteristic of cannabis.

Dronabinol (THC) is primarily metabolized by the cytochrome P450 (CYP450) 2C9 enzyme into 11-hydroxy-THC, and to a lesser degree by CYP3A4 into 7- or 8-hydroxy metabolites (Watanabe et al., 2007). The metabolite 11-hydroxy-THC is pharmacologically active, and polymorphisms of CYP2C9 have been shown to be related to differences in THC response profiles (Sachse-Seeboth et al., 2009), which is an important therapeutic consideration. The exact mechanisms of nabilone metabolism are not known, however it undergoes rapid metabolism to several metabolites including isomeric carbinols (Rubin et al., 1977), and given the long duration of action relative to its rapid metabolism, it has been postulated that some metabolites of nabilone are pharmacologically active.

## 4. Clinical evidence

### 4.1 Self-medication with cannabis

Despite the difficulties of obtaining reliable data, epidemiological studies have found that people with conditions varying from chronic pain, multiple sclerosis (MS), and spinal cord injury sometimes self-medicate with cannabis (Ware et al., 2002). Because cannabis is a restricted drug, for which both possession and supply are illegal in most countries, these surveys have often tended to come from Canada, where the practice of self-medication with cannabis is most openly tolerated (Ogborne *et al.*, 2000a; Ogborne *et al.*, 2000b), although some data is available from the US, UK, and continental Europe.

In Canadian studies of people with chronic pain, up to 38% of the subjects used cannabis daily , with 58% of those people using cannabis more than once a day (Ware et al., 2003). Consumption of cannabis was between 1 and 5 grams a day, which represents up to approximately 65mg THC per day (Lynch et al., 2006). In the UK, 25% of sufferers of chronic pain surveyed had self-medicated with cannabis (Ware et al., 2005). Woolridge and colleagues (Woolridge et al., 2005) found that among 523 HIV-positive patients, almost 27% reported (in an anonymous questionnaire) that they used cannabis to help with HIV associated pain, and most users reported that they experienced improvements in muscle pain (94%) and neuropathic pain (90%).

Some surveys have suggested that large numbers of patients with MS might self-medicate with cannabis (Clark *et al.*, 2004; Ware *et al.*, 2005). In one survey in the UK, 75 patients with MS were questioned, of which 49 experienced chronic pain. Of these patients, 83.7% had tried cannabis to help treat their condition, and 75.6% reported that it provided some relief for their pain (Chong et al., 2006). In an earlier survey that targeted patients with MS that self-medicated with cannabis, some 95% of respondents reported that cannabis improved chronic pain to their extremities, spasticity, and some other symptoms such as bladder and bowel dysfunction (Consroe et al., 1997).

The use of cannabis to treat HIV related symptoms was assessed by Woolridge and colleagues (Woolridge et al., 2005), who surveyed the use of cannabis in HIV-positive individuals attending a large clinic with an anonymous cross-sectional questionnaire. Of those that responded (n=523) 27% reported that they self-medicated with cannabis. Cannabis was reported by the patients to improve appetite (97%), muscle pain (94%), nausea (93%), nerve pain (90%), and paresthesia (85%), but also anxiety (93%) and depression (86%). However, the survey also found that 47% of the cannabis users reported some degree of memory loss.

People with spinal cord injury are another group where self-medication with cannabis is often reported. At the 1998 International Cannabinoid Research Society meeting Consroe and colleagues (Consroe et al., 1998) reported the results of a survey of 190 people with spinal cord injury who belonged to the Alliance for Cannabis Therapeutics of the US. Of the 106 valid respondents, 70% used cannabis along with other medications, and 82% reported that their symptoms became worse when they stopped using cannabis. Improvements were reported for muscle spasms, bladder control, muscle and phantom pains, headache, parathesia, and even paralysis. In a more recent survey of patients with spinal cord injury in the US (Cardenas *et al.*, 2006), 117 patients were questioned about current and past use of treatments. One in seven patients reported having tried an alternative treatment, with cannabis being the most frequently cited. Cannabis was reported to reduce chronic pain by this group by 6.6 points on an 11 point scale, greater than the degree of relief provided by their opioid medications (6.3 points).

In surveys where medicinal cannabis users were targeted, their reasons for use varied considerably, although pain related conditions often appeared high on the list. Schnelle and colleagues reported the results of an anonymous survey of medicinal cannabis users in Germany, Austria and Switzerland (Schnelle et al., 1999). Out of 128 patients that could be included, 12% used medicinal cannabis for depression, 10.8% for MS, 9% HIV-infection, 6.6% migraine, 6% asthma, 5.4% back pain (and 2.4% disk prolapse), 2.4% spinal cord injury, 3% glaucoma, 3.6% spasticity, and 3% nausea. Other conditions included hepatitis C, sleeping disorders, epilepsy, headache, and alcoholism. In this survey, 72.2% of the patients reported that their symptoms were "much improved" by cannabis. In another study, Swift and colleagues (Swift et al., 2005) published the results of an Australian survey following approval of the trial of medical cannabis by the New South Wales State Government. Anonymous questionnaires from 128 participants revealed self-medication with cannabis for chronic pain (57%), depression (56%), arthritis (35%), nausea (27%) and weight loss (26%). Cannabis was also reported to provide substantial relief for pain, nausea and insomnia (Swift et al., 2005). Overall, Australian medical cannabis users reported considerable relief from their symptoms.

Broad survey data on cannabis use sometimes pool recreational and medicinal users, however, despite differences between patterns and levels of use These studies can therefore tend to record frequency of use rather than amounts and potency, measures that are not precisely relevant to people who are self-medicating. Therefore, informal anecdotal or broad survey data is an unreliable guide as to the typical amounts of cannabis and equivalent THC dosages used by people who are self-medicating.

### 4.2 Clinical case reports

Between surveys and randomized clinical trials are clinical case reports. These are often suggestive of a therapeutic effect, but with low N numbers and often lacking placebo controls, are hard to interpret, and sometimes contradict the results of non-clinical experiments. For example, cannabis has been reported by some doctors to reduce pendular nystagmus (Schon *et al.*, 1999; Dell'Osso, 2000), but careful experimentation with more sensitive instruments appears to show that cannabis has little or no effect on the functioning of the vestibular system in humans (Spector, 1973).

Some of the best case studies are controlled experiments, albeit with an N of 1, and include controls consisting of placebos or other drugs. For example, in a study of patient with chronic pain from Mediterranean fever, it was found that the patient significantly increased morphine administration when during periods in the study when he was given a placebo instead of 50 mg THC (Holdcroft et al., 1997). In another study, a single patient with spinal cord injury was treated with either oral THC (5 mg), codeine (50 mg), or a placebo in a double blind trial (Maurer et al., 1990). The study found that THC had a similar analgesic effect to codeine when compared with the placebo, and furthermore that THC reduced spasticity.

Although small clinical case studies and experiments continue to appear in the literature, and although they are of enormous value in indicating valuable directions for more intensive clinical research, the evidence base for the use of cannabinoid therapeutics is rapidly becoming dominated by larger scale clinical trials. For good compilations of clinical observation and anecdote, together with the best clinical trial data of the time and expert interpretation, three publications all released in 1997 by the British Medical Association (BMA) (BMA, 1997), the US National Institutes of Health (NIH) (Bethesda, 1997), and the American Medical Association (AMA) (*Report of the Council on Scientific Affairs to AMA House of Delegates on Medical Marijuana.*, 1997) are authoritative. Additional compilations of patient and doctor testimony can be found in Iversen (Iversen, 2000).

### 4.3 Randomized clinical trials

#### 4.3.1 Acute pain

Campbell et al. (Campbell et al., 2001) reviewed controlled clinical trials, and found that in two trials of acute pain, THC or analogues at tolerable doses were no more effective than codeine, despite increased psychoactivity . Similarly, smoked cannabis was shown to be ineffective in models of experimental acute pain in healthy volunteers, and actually appeared to increase pain sensitivity at higher doses (Hill *et al.*, 1974; Wallace *et al.*, 2007). While this suggests that cannabinoids have minimal efficacy in treating acute nociceptive pain, research in to the use of cannabinoids as adjuvants to opiates for acute pain continues (Greenwald *et al.*, 2000; Buggy *et al.*, 2003; Naef *et al.*, 2003). At least one clinical study has found that THC interacts with morphine to reduce the emotional component of pain (Roberts et al., 2006). Adjuvant therapy would be an attractive therapeutic option due to the adverse effects of opioids when administered at therapeutic doses. Morphine and other opioids cause a number of unwanted and often dose limiting effects, such as constipation, respiratory depression, drowsiness, lack of awareness, and even opioid induced hyperalgesia.

#### 4.3.2 Neuropathic pain

Ashton and Milligan (Ashton *et al.*, 2008) reviewed clinical trials on cannabinoid treatment of neuropathic pain, and found that 15 studies from a total of 18 demonstrated a moderate beneficial effect from cannabinoid treatment.

Wade et al. (Wade et al., 2003) tested whether cannabis extracts (THC, cannabidiol, or Sativex) could treat neurogenic pain and spasm that were intractable to conventional treatment. Pain relief from the drugs was significantly greater than from the placebo. Notcutt et al. (Notcutt et al., 2004) reported that the same three drugs were effective treatments for neuropathic pain, with a side effect profile similar to that for other psychoactive drugs for chronic pain. Berman et al. (Berman et al., 2004) found that Sativex and GW-2000-02 (a cannabis extract containing mostly THC; GW Pharmaceuticals) reduced pain from brachial plexus avulsion for patients with pain refractory to other analgesics, while Sativex has shown further promise in treating allodynia in neuropathic pain syndromes of varying origin (Nurmikko et al., 2007). Pinsger et al. (Pinsger et al., 2006), and Berlach et al. (Berlach et al., 2006) have both tested whether nabilone can control chronic pain, and found a statistically significant decrease in pain, with side effects generally mild. Ajulemic acid, a synthetic analogue of an active metabolite of THC, was found to reduce neuropathic pain in a study by Kaarst et al. (Karst et al., 2003). The results of the study were further extended by Salim et al. (Salim et al., 2005), who calculated that for a clinically relevant 30% reduction in pain, NNT values were 2.14 and 5.29 in two subgroups of patients.

Clinical trials of cannabinoids in multiple sclerosis induced pain are similarly positive. Svendsen et al. (Svendsen et al., 2004) found that pain was reduced by dronabinol in patients with multiple sclerosis related central pain. Nabilone was tested in multiple sclerosis by Wissel et al. (Wissel et al., 2006) who found that pain was reduced by nabilone, but not placebo. A trial of Sativex for the treatment of patients with multiple sclerosis and refractory neuropathic pain by Rog et al. (Rog et al., 2005), found that Sativex relieved pain and was mostly well tolerated. Wade et al. (Wade et al., 2006), in a follow up open-label study to the earlier placebo-controlled trial (Wade et al., 2004) found that mean pain scores were reduced over a 6 week placebo-controlled trial period and then were reduced in the open label study to 40-50% of the baseline scores by weeks 10-26. In the UK, the "Cannabinoids in Multiple Sclerosis (CAMS)" trial compared cannabis extract (Cannador) and dronabinol with placebo (Zajicek et al., 2003). Pain was significantly improved by treatment with either cannabinoid preparation over placebo. Following the main study there was a follow-up double-blinded trial for 12 months (Zajicek et al., 2005), and pain was again relieved to a greater degree in cannabinoid groups over the placebo group.

Two other pain syndromes, HIV-related pain and fibromyalgia deserve special note. Smoked cannabis was found to significantly reduce HIV-induced neuropathic pain by (Abrams et al., 2007), and fibromyalgia-related pain has now been found to be significantly reduced by THC analogues in a number of clinical studies (Schley *et al.*, 2006; Wood *et al.*, 2007; Skrabek *et al.*, 2008).

Clinical evidence for the efficacy of cannabinoids in the treatment of neuropathic pain has not all been positive, and several trials have reported a lack of efficacy. Two of these trials, by Claremont-Gnamien et al. (Clermont-Gnamien et al., 2002) and Attall et al. (Attal et al., 2004), used oral dronabinol, but lacked placebo-controls. In a well controlled study, another report found that nabilone performed poorly compared with dihydrocodeine in treating neuropathic pain of varying origins (Frank et al., 2008). Despite the efficacy of Sativex in treating painful neuropathies (Nurmikko et al., 2007), a recent study in patients suffering painful diabetic neuropathy has been disappointing, with Sativex having no greater effect at relieving pain than placebo (Selvarajah et al., 2010). Similarly , Wade et al. (Wade et al.,

2004) failed to find a beneficial effect on multiple sclerosis induced pain using Sativex. In this instance, Iskedjian et al. (Iskedjian et al., 2007) noted that the placebo effect was unusually large, and patients had unrestricted access to other analgesics. Arguably if Sativex was actually effective in the trial, patients receiving the placebo would initially experience more pain, but then take more of the other analgesics, increasing the apparent pain reduction in the placebo group. This is feasible, as in one case report, a patient with chronic pain increased use of morphine during periods when he was given a placebo instead of THC (Holdcroft et al., 1997).

### 4.3.3 Secondary outcomes

Sleep is also an essential aspect of quality of life, and patients with chronic pain often have difficulty sleeping. Sleep disturbance is itself disturbing and unpleasant, and lack of sleep contributes to fatigue during waking hours. Insomnia is generally treated with central nervous system depressants, which have a number of problems with long term use, including the development of tolerance and dependence, rebound anxiety and insomnia (as well as more severe withdrawal effects), and problems with cognition. Cannabinoids have soporific effects, and the possibility that cannabinoids can help improve sleep when given to patients with chronic pain has been the subject of clinical trials, generally as a secondary outcome measure. In particular, Russo and colleagues (Russo et al., 2007) reviewed the effects of either Sativex in nine clinical trials where sleep disturbance, duration and/or quality was recorded as a secondary outcome measure. The primary outcome measures of these trials were effects on pain, symptoms of multiple sclerosis, and symptoms of arthritis. Seven out of nine trials found that sleep was improved in patients receiving Sativex compared to patients receiving placebo.

### 4.4 Assessing the evidence

In 1997 the British Medical Association reviewed 8 clinical studies (BMA, 1997) and concluded that cannabinoids have a role as adjuvant analgesics for pain conditions refractory to standard drugs. Also in 1997, similar conclusions were made in reports by the American Medical Association (*Report of the Council on Scientific Affairs to AMA House of Delegates on Medical Marijuana.*, 1997) and the US National Institutes of Health (Bethesda, 1997). Despite this, it is clear to see that the evidence from clinical trials is not consistent, with some but not all trials showing a moderate effect on neuropathic pain from cannabinoid treatment.

The inconsistency of the evidence may be partly due to the inconsistency of the quality of the randomized clinical trials. The risk of unblinding of subjects to treatment has been high in a number of trials; some subjects had prior exposure to cannabis or even cannabinoid drugs in open phases of the trials. Another possible explanation for the inconsistency of evidence could be the heterogeneity of pain syndromes and outcome measures across trials. Much of the evidence for antinociceptive effects in neuropathic pain comes from studies primarily aimed at assessing spasticity in multiple sclerosis, or neuropathic pain of varying origin and severity. In conditions with severe neuropathies, cannabinoids at tolerable doses may be less efficacious. This is illustrated by the disparity between the positive results of Nurmikko et al. (Nurmikko et al., 2007), who report Sativex was efficacious in the treatment of neuropathic pain of different origins, and those of Selvarajah et al., (Selvarajah et al.,

2010), who report no effect of Sativex on painful poly-neuropathy. This issue is discussed in a major recent systematic review of drug treatment for neuropathic pain (Finnerup et al., 2010). In it, Finnerup et al. concluded that cannabinoids have a small effect on central pain in multiple sclerosis, mixed neuropathic pain and in peripheral neuropathic pain, but not in painful poly-neuropathy.

A meta-analysis published in 2007 (Iskedjian et al., 2007) reported that cannabinoids are useful for neuropathic pain. Iskedjian et al. (Iskedjian et al., 2007) analysed data from 6 published studies and additional unpublished data from GW Pharmaceuticals. Sativex decreased pain by 1.7 +/- 0.7 points ($p = 0.018$) on an 11-point scale; cannabidiol by 1.5 +/- 0.7 points ($p = 0.044$); dronabinol by 1.5 +/- 0.6 points ($p = 0.013$). Pooling the 3 drugs together, pain reduction was 1.6 +/- 0.4 points ($p < 0.001$) for the cannabinoid group, in contrast to 0.8 +/- 0.4 points ($p = 0.023$) for the placebo. Average baseline scores in the trials were around 50-70% of the maximum possible pain, thus a cannabinoid-induced 1.6 point reduction on a 11-point scale would be equate to an approximately 24% reduction in pain. An important consideration in analysing this clinical data is that many trials have studied patients with pain refractory to conventional treatment, and concomitant analgesia is the norm, thus some part of the analgesia provided by the cannabinoids may be masked. In addition, most trials only tested for pain reduction for a short time; Isdekjian et al. (Iskedjian et al., 2007) found that pain reduction was doubled in subjects receiving a cannabis-based medicinal extract (CBME) at 6-10 weeks compared with earlier times, an approximate halving of baseline pain scores. It was further suggested that the patients in the drug group who showed improvement for pain could be "cannabinoid responders" who have greater than the average pain relief.

## 5. Safety and tolerability

### 5.1 Adverse events

In clinical trials using cannabinoids, adverse side effects are dose dependent, and appear to vary in intensity from trial to trial, and between individuals within trials. Possible side effects include euphoria, dysphoria, anxiety, depersonalisation, sedation and drowsiness, distorted perception, mental clouding, memory impairment, impairment on cognitively demanding tasks, fragmentation of thoughts, and even hallucinations. Cannabinoids also stimulate appetite, and in some contexts this might possibly be considered an undesired effect; though it is an effect that is actively sought when cannabinoids are used to stimulate weight gain in patients suffering from wasting after HIV infection or chemotherapy. Acute cannabis toxicity can cause psychotic episodes involving delusions and paranoia. With respect to motor function, cannabis can cause hypermotility (increased motor activity, movement) followed by lethargy, lack of coordination or ataxia, muscle twitches, tremors and weakness, and problems speaking (dysarthia). Pregnant women should avoid cannabinoids, as this been linked to the impairment of fetal development (Hurd *et al.*, 2005; Huizink *et al.*, 2006), even though the evidence for this is inconsistent (Chiriboga, 2003).

Most clinical trials discussed earlier also contain data on adverse effects. These are mostly minor, and virtually all the trials describe the drug as "well tolerated". The most common side effects reported in the trials are drowsiness, ataxia, euphoria and dizziness. At higher doses, dissociation and distorted perception are infrequently reported. For example, in the trials carried out by Berman et al. (Berman et al., 2004) and Rog et al. (Rog et al., 2005), approximately 25 mg of THC was used, and adverse effects were mild to moderate, and usually spontaneously resolved. In both trials the most common side effects were dizziness and drowsiness. In the Rog et al. (Rog et al., 2005) trial, 53% of patients experienced at least one episode of dizziness, 1 out of 34 patients experienced drowsiness ("somnolence") and 1 out of 34 experienced dissociation and ataxia ("feeling drunk"). It is important to note that this trial (which is typical) recorded at least one minor adverse event for 88.2% of patients on the drug, but to put this in context, the figure is 68.8% for patients taking the placebo.

As neuropathic pain is a condition requiring long term treatment, it is important to assess the adverse effects of any treatment over an appropriate time course. Wade et al. (Wade et al., 2006) and Zajicek et al. (Zajicek et al., 2005) both reported on the long term effects of THC medication in pain conditions. Wade et al. (Wade et al., 2006) extended a placebo controlled acute trial in multiple sclerosis patients, and investigated long term Sativex use in an open label trial. They noted that adverse effects were mild in most cases, and the few serious events recorded (seizure, gastroenteritis, pneumonia) could not be definitively linked to Sativex use, as patients were taking other medications, and multiple sclerosis in itself is a risk factor for some of the recorded events. Similarly, Zajicek et al. (Zajicek et al., 2005) extended a placebo controlled trial of dronabinol and cannabis extract (Cannador) in multiple sclerosis patients, and recorded adverse events for a year. Unlike the Wade et al. follow up, the design of the study allowed comparison of cannabinoid treatment with an inactive placebo. While minor and serious adverse events were reported in the cannabinoid groups, incidence rates were comparable with placebo (Zajicek et al., 2005). Overall both studies conclude that in general, adverse effects were mild, and long term cannabinoid treatment was well tolerated.

### 5.2 Tolerance and dependence

In studies dealing with self medication with cannabis, it is difficult to accurately calculate equivalent doses of THC, as frequency, amount, and potency of smoked cannabis leaf are highly variable between users. A recent study with 30 subjects in Canada found that people who used cannabis to treat themselves for chronic pain used between 1 and 5 grams of cannabis a day, with an average of 2.5 grams/day (Lynch et al., 2006). The THC content in cannabis cigarettes usually ranges between 1.5 to 3.7%, so smoking 2.5g per day translates into a daily intake of 38 to 93 mg of THC. As only 10 to 25% of the THC in smoked cannabis leaf will be absorbed into the bloodstream (Adams *et al.*, 1996), this equates to 3.8 to 23 mg of THC per day. The other systematic source of data on amounts of THC that will be sought by people seeking relief from chronic pain comes from clinical trials where the patients are allowed to "self-titrate". This is where the patient has *ad libitum* access to the drug (within an upper limit), and takes the drug as required. In this way, the patient finds a balance between the desired and undesired effects to fit their individual needs. In these self-titrating trials, 25 mg of THC was a typical amount of the drug that was taken during a day. Therefore, there appears to be a reasonable correlation between the amounts of THC that people seek from self-medication with cannabis, and from purified extracts in clinical trials.

People who self-titrate, or self-medicate for THC may raise the dose that they seek over time, because they can become tolerant to the analgesic effects of THC (Association, 1997; Lichtman *et al.*, 2005), and thus seek higher amounts to relieve their pain. At the same time, tolerance also occurs to adverse effects, such as drowsiness and sedation. With respect to euphoria and minor adverse effects, moderate and heavy users of cannabis do develop tolerance (i.e., a decreased response to the drug) (Lichtman *et al.*, 2005). In one study, heavy users smoked an average 5.7 grams of cannabis a day, and showed a progressive decline in ratings of intoxication (Babor et al., 1975).

Cannabis dependence is a recognised syndrome under DSM-IV criteria, and has been the subject of a number of epidemiological studies (e.g., (Fergusson *et al.*, 2003; Boden *et al.*, 2006)). The official advice seems to indicate that cannabis dependence is not prevalent. The UM MRHA 2007 report on Sativex states that only 1% of cannabis users develop dependence on the drug. The prescription data sheets for Cesamet and Marinol state that in clinical trials of these formulations in patient populations, patients experienced no withdrawal symptoms, despite a 5 month trial in the case of Marinol. Both data sheets, however, point to an abstinence syndrome in healthy volunteers after the cessation of large daily doses of THC (200 mg), administered over 12 - 16 days. Withdrawal symptoms included some distress, sleep disturbances and autonomic hyperactivity, lasting for 48 hours after drug cessation.

## 6. Future drug development

One of the limiting factors for the widespread clinical use of cannabinoids is adverse psychoactivity. As discussed earlier, this is caused exclusively by activation of CB1 receptors in the central nervous system. One important aim of research into cannabinoid receptors as therapeutic targets is to obtain ligands with clinically useful effects, but without (or at least minimizing) the psychoactive unwanted effects. The chronic pain relieving properties are thought to be mediated via activation of not only central CB1 receptors, but also spinal and peripheral CB1 and CB2 receptors. Recent cannabinoid drug development has attempted to exploit the apparent redundancy of the cannabinoid system in pain, developing ligands selective for non-psychoactive or peripheral cannabinoid receptors.

Because of the distinct distributions and physiological functions of CB1 and CB2, there has been intensive research into developing ligands specific for a particular receptor, particularly the "non-psychoactive" CB2 receptor. HU-308 is a highly selective bicyclic CB2-agonist, related to WIN55,212-2 and JWH-133, with a 440-fold selectivity for CB2 over CB1 (Hanus et al., 1999). At the time of writing, HU-308 has restricted availability, and is being intensively studied by several research groups for its potential therapeutic potential. Another highly selective CB2 agonist, GW405833, has been synthesised (Valenzano et al., 2005), and is also a derivative of WIN55,212-2. Crucially, although this compound has only 80-fold selectivity for the CB2 receptor over the CB1 receptor in rats, it has a 1200-fold selectivity for CB2 over CB1 in humans. GW405833 is a partial agonist at CB2 (Kearn et al., 1999). Preclinical research into these compounds has been promising, although clinical translation has been less so. GlaxoSmithKline tested GW842166, a potent CB2 agonist, and found it to be highly efficacious in an animal model of inflammatory pain. In the clinic, however, this compound had no effect on acute dental pain compared to placebo in a paradigm where 800 mg ibuprofen was efficacious (Ostenfeld et al., 2011). This said, it must be questioned why a condition of acute pain was chosen for clinical testing in this instance, as cannabinoids have typically been more efficacious in chronic pain conditions.

Alternatively, the selective targeting of peripheral cannabinoid receptors would also circumvent unfavourable psychoactivity. AstraZeneca have been conducting preclinical and clinical trials with several peripherally restricted cannabinoid agonists with mixed results. Preclinical trials with AZ11713908 (Yu et al., 2010) and AZD1940 (Groblewski *et al.*, 2010b) indicated antinociceptive efficacy in animal models of inflammatory and neuropathic pain, and minimal CNS penetration. In clinical trials, however, AZD1940 reportedly had no effect on acute dental pain, or chronic back pain (Groblewski *et al.*, 2010a).

## 7. Conclusions

Cannabis is widely used by people suffering from neuropathic pain, with many users reporting pain relieving effects. In more quantitative analyses, cannabinoids appear to have a moderate efficacy in the treatment of chronic and neuropathic pain of varying origin, with adverse effects and dependence risk minimal when compared with traditional analgesics, especially opioids. Despite a lack of efficacy in every neuropathic condition, and dose limiting adverse effects of these compounds, there appears to be a large body of evidence supporting a continued role of cannabinoids as analgesics in some instances, especially in patients refractory to current treatments. The development of more efficacious and well tolerated drugs in this class will enable a more widespread application these pharmacotherapeutics in neuropathic pain.

## 8. References

Abrams, DI, Jay, CA, Shade, SB, Vizoso, H, Reda, H, Press, S, Kelly, ME, Rowbotham, MC, Petersen, KL. (2007). Cannabis in painful HIV-associated sensory neuropathy: a randomized placebo-controlled trial. *Neurology,* Vol. 68, No. 7, pp. (515-521)

Adams, IB, Martin, BR. (1996). Cannabis: pharmacology and toxicology in animals and humans. *Addiction,* Vol. 91, No. 11, pp. (1585-1614)

Agarwal, N, Pacher, P, Tegeder, I, Amaya, F, Constantin, CE, Brenner, GJ, Rubino, T, Michalski, CW, Marsicano, G, Monory, K, Mackie, K, Marian, C, Batkai, S, Parolaro, D, Fischer, MJ, Reeh, P, Kunos, G, Kress, M, Lutz, B, Woolf, CJ, Kuner, R. (2007). Cannabinoids mediate analgesia largely via peripheral type 1 cannabinoid receptors in nociceptors. *Nat Neurosci,* Vol. 10, No. 7, pp. (870-879)

Ashton, JC, Milligan, ED. (2008). Cannabinoids for the treatment of neuropathic pain: clinical evidence. *Curr Opin Investig Drugs,* Vol. 9, No. 1, pp. (65-75)

Association, BM (1997) *Therapeutic uses of Cannabis.* Harwood Academic Publishers, Amsterdam.

Attal, N, Brasseur, L, Guirimand, D, Clermond-Gnamien, S, Atlami, S, Bouhassira, D. (2004). Are oral cannabinoids safe and effective in refractory neuropathic pain? *Eur J Pain,* Vol. 8, No. 2, pp. (173-177)

Babor, TF, Mendelson, JH, Greenberg, I, Kuehnle, JC. (1975). Marijuana consumption and tolerance to physiological and subjective effects. *Arch Gen Psychiatry,* Vol. 32, No. 12, pp. (1548-1552)

Benito, C, Nunez, E, Tolon, RM, Carrier, EJ, Rabano, A, Hillard, CJ, Romero, J. (2003). Cannabinoid CB2 receptors and fatty acid amide hydrolase are selectively overexpressed in neuritic plaque-associated glia in Alzheimer's disease brains. *J Neurosci,* Vol. 23, No. 35, pp. (11136-11141)

Berlach, DM, Shir, Y, Ware, MA. (2006). Experience with the synthetic cannabinoid nabilone in chronic noncancer pain. *Pain Med,* Vol. 7, No. 1, pp. (25-29)

Berman, JS, Symonds, C, Birch, R. (2004). Efficacy of two cannabis based medicinal extracts for relief of central neuropathic pain from brachial plexus avulsion: results of a randomised controlled trial. *Pain,* Vol. 112, No. 3, pp. (299-306)

Bethesda, MD (1997) *Report on the Medical Uses of Marijuana.*: National Institutes of Health.

BMA (1997) *Therapeutic uses of cannabis.* Harwood Academic Publishers: Amsterdam.

Boden, JM, Fergusson, DM, Horwood, LJ. (2006). Illicit drug use and dependence in a New Zealand birth cohort. *Aust N Z J Psychiatry,* Vol. 40, No. 2, pp. (156-163)

Buggy, DJ, Toogood, L, Maric, S, Sharpe, P, Lambert, DG, Rowbotham, DJ. (2003). Lack of analgesic efficacy of oral delta-9-tetrahydrocannabinol in postoperative pain. *Pain,* Vol. 106, No. 1-2, pp. (169-172)

Burns, TL, Ineck, JR. (2006). Cannabinoid analgesia as a potential new therapeutic option in the treatment of chronic pain. *Ann Pharmacother,* Vol. 40, No. 2, pp. (251-260)

Cabral, G, Marciano-Cabral, F. (2005). Cannabinoid receptors in microglia of the central nervous system: immune functional relevance. *J Leukoc Biol.,* Vol. 78, No. 6, pp. (1192-1197)

Campbell, FA, Tramer, MR, Carroll, D, Reynolds, DJ, Moore, RA, McQuay, HJ. (2001). Are cannabinoids an effective and safe treatment option in the management of pain? A qualitative systematic review. *Bmj,* Vol. 323, No. 7303, pp. (13-16)

Cardenas, DD, Jensen, MP. (2006). Treatments for chronic pain with spinal cord injury: A survey study. *J Spinal Cord Med.,* Vol. 29, No. 2, pp. (109-117)

Chiriboga, CA. (2003). Fetal alcohol and drug effects. *Neurologist,* Vol. 9, No. 6, pp. (267-279)

Chong, MS, Wolff, K, Wise, K, Tanton, C, Winstock, A, Silber, E. (2006). Cannabis use in patients with multiple sclerosis. *Mult Scler,* Vol. 12, No. 5, pp. (646-651)

Clark, AJ, Ware, MA, Yazer, E, Murray, TJ, Lynch, ME. (2004). Patterns of cannabis use among patients with multiple sclerosis. *Neurology,* Vol. 62, No. 11, pp. (2098-2100)

Clarke, RC, Watson, DP (2002) Botany of Natural Cannabis Medicines. In: *Cannabis and Cannabinoids: Pharmacology and Toxicology and Therapeutic Potential,* Grotenhermen, MD, Russo, E (eds), pp 3-13. New York: The Hawthorn Integrative Healing Press.

Clermont-Gnamien, S, Atlani, S, Attal, N, Le Mercier, F, Guirimand, F, Brasseur, L. (2002). [The therapeutic use of D9-tetrahydrocannabinol (dronabinol) in refractory neuropathic pain]. *Presse Med,* Vol. 31, No. 39 Pt 1, pp. (1840-1845)

Compton, DR, Johnson, MR, Melvin, LS, Martin, BR. (1992). Pharmacological profile of a series of bicyclic cannabinoid analogs: classification as cannabimimetic agents. *J Pharmacol Exp Ther.,* Vol. 260, No. 1, pp. (201-209)

Consroe, P, Musty, R, Rein, J, Tillery, W, Pertwee, R. (1997). The perceived effects of smoked cannabis on patients with multiple sclerosis. *Eur Neurol.,* Vol. 38, No. pp. (44-48.)

Consroe, P, Tillery, W, Rein, J, Musty, RE. (1998). Reported marijuana effects in patients with spinal cord injury., *International Cannabinoid Research Society, Symposium on Cannabinoids,* Burlington, Vermont.,

Cravatt, BF, Giang, DK, Mayfield, SP, Boger, DL, Lerner, RA, Gilula, NB. (1996). Molecular characterization of an enzyme that degrades neuromodulatory fatty-acid amides. *Nature.,* Vol. 384, No. 6604, pp. (83-87)

Cronin, CM, Sallan, SE, Gelber, R, Lucas, VS, Laszlo, J. (1981). Antiemetic effect of intramuscular levonantradol in patients receiving anticancer chemotherapy. *J Clin Pharmacol,* Vol. 21, No. 8-9 Suppl, pp. (43S-50S)

Dell'Osso, LF. (2000). Suppression of pendular nystagmus by smoking cannabis in a patient with multiple sclerosis. *Neurology,* Vol. 54, No. 11, pp. (2190-2191)

Devane, WA, Dysarz, FA, 3rd, Johnson, MR, Melvin, LS, Howlett, AC. (1988). Determination and characterization of a cannabinoid receptor in rat brain. *Mol Pharmacol.,* Vol. 34, No. 5, pp. (605-613.)

Devane, WA, Hanus, L, Breuer, A, Pertwee, RG, Stevenson, LA, Griffin, G, Gibson, D, Mandelbaum, A, Etinger, A, Mechoulam, R. (1992). Isolation and structure of a brain constituent that binds to the cannabinoid receptor. *Science.,* Vol. 258, No. 5090, pp. (1946-1949.)

Di Marzo, V. (2006a). A brief history of cannabinoid and endocannabinoid pharmacology as inspired by the work of British scientists. *Trends Pharmacol Sci.,* Vol. 27, No. 3, pp. (134-140)

Di Marzo, V. (2006b). A brief history of cannabinoid and endocannabinoid pharmacology as inspired by the work of British scientists. *Trends Pharmacol Sci,* Vol. 27, No. 3, pp. (134-140)

Dinh, TP, Carpenter, D, Leslie, FM, Freund, TF, Katona, I, Sensi, SL, Kathuria, S, Piomelli, D. (2002). Brain monoglyceride lipase participating in endocannabinoid inactivation. *Proc Natl Acad Sci U S A.,* Vol. 99, No. 16, pp. (10819-10824)

Elphick, MR, Egertova, M. (2001). The neurobiology and evolution of cannabinoid signalling. *Philos Trans R Soc Lond B Biol Sci.,* Vol. 356, No. 1407, pp. (381-408.)

Fergusson, DM, Horwood, LJ, Lynskey, MT, Madden, PA. (2003). Early reactions to cannabis predict later dependence. *Arch Gen Psychiatry,* Vol. 60, No. 10, pp. (1033-1039)

Finnerup, NB, Sindrup, SH, Jensen, TS. (2010). The evidence for pharmacological treatment of neuropathic pain. *Pain,* Vol. 150, No. 3, pp. (573-581)

Frank, B, Serpell, MG, Hughes, J, Matthews, JN, Kapur, D. (2008). Comparison of analgesic effects and patient tolerability of nabilone and dihydrocodeine for chronic neuropathic pain: randomised, crossover, double blind study. *Bmj,* Vol. 336, No. 7637, pp. (199-201)

Frankhauser, M (2002) History of Cannabis in Western Medicine. In: *Cannabis and Cannabinoids: Pharmacology, Toxicology, and Therapeutic Potential.,* Grotenhermen, F, Russo, E (eds). New York: The Haworth Integrative Healing Press.

Galiegue, S, Mary, S, Marchand, J, Dussossoy, D, Carriere, D, Carayon, P, Bouaboula, M, Shire, D, Le Fur, G, Casellas, P. (1995). Expression of central and peripheral cannabinoid receptors in human immune tissues and leukocyte subpopulations. *Eur J Biochem.,* Vol. 232, No. 1, pp. (54-61)

Gerard, CM, Mollereau, C, Vassart, G, Parmentier, M. (1991). Molecular cloning of a human cannabinoid receptor which is also expressed in testis. *Biochem J,* Vol. 279, No. 1, pp. (129-134)

Glass, M, Dragunow, M, Faull, RL. (1997). Cannabinoid receptors in the human brain: a detailed anatomical and quantitative autoradiographic study in the fetal, neonatal and adult human brain. *Neuroscience,* Vol. 77, No. 2, pp. (299-318.)

Gong, JP, Onaivi, ES, Ishiguro, H, Liu, QR, Tagliaferro, PA, Brusco, A, Uhl, GR. (2006). Cannabinoid CB2 receptors: immunohistochemical localization in rat brain. *Brain Res,* Vol. 1071, No. 1, pp. (10-23)

Greenwald, MK, Stitzer, ML. (2000). Antinociceptive, subjective and behavioral effects of smoked marijuana in humans. *Drug Alcohol Depend,* Vol. 59, No. 3, pp. (261-275)

Griffin, G, Tao, Q, Abood, ME. (2000). Cloning and pharmacological characterization of the rat CB(2) cannabinoid receptor. *J Pharmacol Exp Ther,* Vol. 292, No. 3, pp. (886-894)

Groblewski, T, Karlsten, R, Segerdhal, M, Kalliomaki, J, Jonzon, B, Bielenstein, M, Cebers, G, Swedberg, M, Annas, A, Christoph, G, Tellefors, P, Stahle, L, Bouw, R, Fagerholm,

U, Berg, A, Butler, S, O'Malley, M, Anstren, G. (2010a). Peripherally-acting CB1-CB2 agonists for pain: do they still hold promise?, *Proceedings of the 20th annual symposium of the international cannabinoid research society,* Lund, Sweden, July 2010.

Groblewski, T, Yu, XH, Laessard, E, St-Onge, S, Yang, H, Panetta, R, Cao, CQ, Swedberg, M, Cebers, G, Nyberg, S, Schou, M, Halldin, C, Gulyas, B, Varnas, K, Walpole, C, Payza, K, Perkins, M, Ducharme, J. (2010b). Pre-clinical pharmacological properties of novel peripherally-acting CB1-CB2 agonists, *Proceedings of the 20th annual symposium of the international cannabinoid research society,* Lund, Sweden, July 2010.

Hanus, L, Breuer, A, Tchilibon, S, Shiloah, S, Goldenberg, D, Horowitz, M, Pertwee, RG, Ross, RA, Mechoulam, R, Fride, E. (1999). HU-308: a specific agonist for CB(2), a peripheral cannabinoid receptor. *Proc Natl Acad Sci U S A,* Vol. 96, No. 25, pp. (14228-14233)

Herkenham, M, Lynn, AB, Little, MD, Johnson, MR, Melvin, LS, de Costa, BR, Rice, KC. (1990a). Cannabinoid receptor localization in brain. *Proc Natl Acad Sci U S A.,* Vol. 87, No. 5, pp. (1932-1936)

Herkenham, M, Lynn, AB, Little, MD, Johnson, MR, Melvin, LS, de Costa, BR, Rice, KC. (1990b). Cannabinoid receptor localization in brain. *Proc Natl Acad Sci U S A,* Vol. 87, No. 5, pp. (1932-1936)

Hill, SY, Schwin, R, Goodwin, DW, Powell, BJ. (1974). Marihuana and pain. *J Pharmacol Exp Ther,* Vol. 188, No. 2, pp. (415-418)

Holdcroft, A, Smith, M, Jacklin, A, Hodgson, H, Smith, B, Newton, M, Evans, F. (1997). Pain relief with oral cannabinoids in familial Mediterranean fever. *Anaesthesia,* Vol. 52, No. 5, pp. (483-486)

Huffman, JW. (2005). CB2 receptor ligands. *Mini Rev Med Chem.,* Vol. 5, No. 7, pp. (641-649.)

Huizink, AC, Mulder, EJ. (2006). Maternal smoking, drinking or cannabis use during pregnancy and neurobehavioral and cognitive functioning in human offspring. *Neurosci Biobehav Rev,* Vol. 30, No. 1, pp. (24-41)

Hurd, YL, Wang, X, Anderson, V, Beck, O, Minkoff, H, Dow-Edwards, D. (2005). Marijuana impairs growth in mid-gestation fetuses. *Neurotoxicol Teratol,* Vol. 27, No. 2, pp. (221-229)

Huskey, A. (2006). Cannabinoids in cancer pain management. *J Pain Palliat Care Pharmacother,* Vol. 20, No. 3, pp. (43-46)

Hutcheon, AW, Palmer, JB, Soukop, M, Cunningham, D, McArdle, C, Welsh, J, Stuart, F, Sangster, G, Kaye, S, Charlton, D, et al. (1983). A randomised multicentre single blind comparison of a cannabinoid anti-emetic (levonantradol) with chlorpromazine in patients receiving their first cytotoxic chemotherapy. *Eur J Cancer Clin Oncol,* Vol. 19, No. 8, pp. (1087-1090)

Iskedjian, M, Bereza, B, Gordon, A, Piwko, C, Einarson, TR. (2007). Meta-analysis of cannabis based treatments for neuropathic and multiple sclerosis-related pain. *Curr Med Res Opin,* Vol. 23, No. 1, pp. (17-24)

Iversen, L (2000) *The Science of Marijuana.* Oxford University Press: Oxford.

Izzo, AA, Mascolo, N, Capasso, F. (2001). The gastrointestinal pharmacology of cannabinoids. *Curr Opin Pharmacol.,* Vol. 1, No. 6, pp. (597-603)

Jain, AK, Ryan, JR, McMahon, FG, Smith, G. (1981). Evaluation of intramuscular levonantradol and placebo in acute postoperative pain. *J Clin Pharmacol,* Vol. 21, No. pp. (320S-326S)

Karst, M, Salim, K, Burstein, S, Conrad, I, Hoy, L, Schneider, U. (2003). Analgesic Effect of the Synthetic Cannabinoid CT-3 on Chronic Neuropathic Pain. *JAMA,* Vol. 290, No. 13, pp. (1757-1762)

Kearn, CS, Greenberg, MJ, DiCamelli, R, Kurzawa, K, Hillard, CJ. (1999). Relationships between ligand affinities for the cerebellar cannabinoid receptor CB1 and the induction of GDP/GTP exchange. *J Neurochem.,* Vol. 72, No. 6, pp. (2379-2387)

Lees, G, Dougalis, A. (2004). Differential effects of the sleep-inducing lipid oleamide and cannabinoids on the induction of long-term potentiation in the CA1 neurons of the rat hippocampus in vitro. *Brain Res.,* Vol. 997, No. 1, pp. (1-14)

Lichtman, AH, Martin, BR. (2005). Cannabinoid tolerance and dependence. *Handb Exp Pharmacol,* Vol. No. 168, pp. (691-717)

Lynch, ME, Young, J, Clark, AJ. (2006). A case series of patients using medicinal marihuana for management of chronic pain under the Canadian Marihuana Medical Access Regulations. *J Pain Symptom Manage,* Vol. 32, No. 5, pp. (497-501)

Machado Rocha, FC, StÉFano, SC, De CÁSsia Haiek, R, Rosa Oliveira, LMQ, Da Silveira, DX. (2008). Therapeutic use of Cannabis sativa on chemotherapy-induced nausea and vomiting among cancer patients: systematic review and meta-analysis. *European Journal of Cancer Care,* Vol. 17, No. 5, pp. (431-443)

Manzanares, J, Julian, MD, Carrascosa, A. (2006). Current Neuropharmacology. *Role of the Cannabinoid System in Pain Control and Therapeutic Implications for the Management of Acute and Chronic Pain Episodes.,* Vol. 4, No. pp. (239-257)

Maurer, M, Henn, V, Dittrich, A, Hofmann, A. (1990). Delta-9-tetrahydrocannabinol shows antispastic and analgesic effects in a single case double-blind trial. *Eur Arch Psychiatry Clin Neurosci,* Vol. 240, No. 1, pp. (1-4)

Mechoulam, R, Ben-Shabat, S, Hanus, L, Ligumsky, M, Kaminski, NE, Schatz, AR, Gopher, A, Almog, S, Martin, BR, Compton, DR, et al. (1995). Identification of an endogenous 2-monoglyceride, present in canine gut, that binds to cannabinoid receptors. *Biochem Pharmacol.,* Vol. 50, No. 1, pp. (83-90)

Mechoulam, R, Gaoni, Y. (1965). A Total Synthesis of Dl-Delta-1-Tetrahydrocannabinol, the Active Constituent of Hashish. *J Am Chem Soc.,* Vol. 87, No. pp. (3273-3275)

Medicines and Healthcare products Regulatory Agency, U (2007) *Public Information Report on Sativex Oromucosal Spray: UK/H/961/01/DC.*

Munro, S, Thomas, KL, Abu-Shaar, M. (1993). Molecular characterization of a peripheral receptor for cannabinoids. *Nature.,* Vol. 365, No. 6441, pp. (61-65)

Naef, M, Curatolo, M, Petersen-Felix, S, Arendt-Nielsen, L, Zbinden, A, Brenneisen, R. (2003). The analgesic effect of oral delta-9-tetrahydrocannabinol (THC), morphine, and a THC-morphine combination in healthy subjects under experimental pain conditions. *Pain,* Vol. 105, No. 1-2, pp. (79-88)

Njie, YF, Kumar, A, Qiao, Z, Zhong, L, Song, ZH. (2006). Noladin ether acts on trabecular meshwork cannabinoid (CB1) receptors to enhance aqueous humor outflow facility. *Invest Ophthalmol Vis Sci.,* Vol. 47, No. 5, pp. (1999-2005)

Notcutt, W, Price, M, Miller, R, Newport, S, Phillips, C, Simmons, S, Sansom, C. (2004). Initial experiences with medicinal extracts of cannabis for chronic pain: results from 34 'N of 1' studies. *Anaesthesia,* Vol. 59, No. 5, pp. (440-452)

Nurmikko, TJ, Serpell, MG, Hoggart, B, Toomey, PJ, Morlion, BJ, Haines, D. (2007). Sativex successfully treats neuropathic pain characterised by allodynia: a randomised, double-blind, placebo-controlled clinical trial. *Pain,* Vol. 133, No. 1-3, pp. (210-220)

Ogborne, AC, Smart, RG. (2000a). Cannabis users in the general Canadian population. *Subst Use Misuse,* Vol. 35, No. 3, pp. (301-311)

Ogborne, AC, Smart, RG, Adlaf, EM. (2000b). Self-reported medical use of marijuana: a survey of the general population. *Cmaj,* Vol. 162, No. 12, pp. (1685-1686)

Okamoto, Y, Wang, J, Morishita, J, Ueda, N. (2007). Biosynthetic pathways of the endocannabinoid anandamide. *Chem Biodivers,* Vol. 4, No. 8, pp. (1842-1857)

Onaivi, ES, Ishiguro, H, Gong, JP, Patel, S, Perchuk, A, Meozzi, PA, Myers, L, Mora, Z, Tagliaferro, P, Gardner, E, Brusco, A, Akinshola, BE, Liu, QR, Hope, B, Iwasaki, S, Arinami, T, Teasenfitz, L, Uhl, GR. (2006). Discovery of the presence and functional expression of cannabinoid CB2 receptors in brain. *Ann N Y Acad Sci,* Vol. 1074, No. pp. (514-536)

Ostenfeld, T, Price, J, Albanese, M, Bullman, J, Guillard, F, Meyer, I, Leeson, R, Costantin, C, Ziviani, L, Nocini, PF, Milleri, S. (2011). A Randomized, Controlled Study to Investigate the Analgesic Efficacy of Single Doses of the Cannabinoid Receptor-2 Agonist GW842166, Ibuprofen or Placebo in Patients With Acute Pain Following Third Molar Tooth Extraction. *Clin J Pain,* Vol. 27, No. 8, pp. (668-676)

Pacher, P, Batkai, S, Kunos, G. (2006). The endocannabinoid system as an emerging target of pharmacotherapy. *Pharmacol Rev.,* Vol. 58, No. 3, pp. (389-462.)

Park, B, Gibbons, HM, Mitchell, MD, Glass, M. (2003). Identification of the CB1 cannabinoid receptor and fatty acid amide hydrolase (FAAH) in the human placenta. *Placenta.,* Vol. 24, No. 10, pp. (990-995)

Pertwee, RG. (2001). Cannabinoid receptors and pain. *Prog Neurobiol,* Vol. 63, No. 5, pp. (569-611)

Pinsger, M, Schimetta, W, Volc, D, Hiermann, E, Riederer, F, Polz, W. (2006). [Benefits of an add-on treatment with the synthetic cannabinomimetic nabilone on patients with chronic pain--a randomized controlled trial]. *Wien Klin Wochenschr,* Vol. 118, No. 11-12, pp. (327-335)

*Report of the Council on Scientific Affairs to AMA House of Delegates on Medical Marijuana.* (1997). American Medical Association.

Rinaldi-Carmona, M, Barth, F, Heaulme, M, Shire, D, Calandra, B, Congy, C, Martinez, S, Maruani, J, Neliat, G, Caput, D, et al. (1994). SR141716A, a potent and selective antagonist of the brain cannabinoid receptor. *FEBS Lett.,* Vol. 350, No. 2-3, pp. (240-244)

Roberts, JD, Gennings, C, Shih, M. (2006). Synergistic affective analgesic interaction between delta-9-tetrahydrocannabinol and morphine. *Eur J Pharmacol,* Vol. 530, No. 1-2, pp. (54-58)

Robson, P. (2005). Human studies of cannabinoids and medicinal cannabis. *Handb Exp Pharmacol,* Vol. No. 168, pp. (719-756)

Rog, DJ, Nurmikko, TJ, Friede, T, Young, CA. (2005). Randomized, controlled trial of cannabis-based medicine in central pain in multiple sclerosis. *Neurology,* Vol. 65, No. 6, pp. (812-819)

Rubin, A, Lemberger, L, Warrick, P, Crabtree, RE, Sullivan, H, Rowe, H, Obermeyer, BD. (1977). Physiologic disposition of nabilone, a cannabinol derivative, in man. *Clin Pharmacol Ther,* Vol. 22, No. 1, pp. (85-91)

Russo, EB, Guy, GW, Robson, PJ. (2007). Cannabis, pain, and sleep: lessons from therapeutic clinical trials of Sativex, a cannabis-based medicine. *Chem Biodivers,* Vol. 4, No. 8, pp. (1729-1743)

Sachse-Seeboth, C, Pfeil, J, Sehrt, D, Meineke, I, Tzvetkov, M, Bruns, E, Poser, W, Vormfelde, SV, Brockmoller, J. (2009). Interindividual variation in the pharmacokinetics of

Delta9-tetrahydrocannabinol as related to genetic polymorphisms in CYP2C9. *Clin Pharmacol Ther,* Vol. 85, No. 3, pp. (273-276)

Salim, K, Schneider, U, Burstein, S, Hoy, L, Karst, M. (2005). Pain measurements and side effect profile of the novel cannabinoid ajulemic acid. *Neuropharmacology,* Vol. 48, No. 8, pp. (1164-1171)

Schley, M, Legler, A, Skopp, G, Schmelz, M, Konrad, C, Rukwied, R. (2006). Delta-9-THC based monotherapy in fibromyalgia patients on experimentally induced pain, axon reflex flare, and pain relief. *Curr Med Res Opin,* Vol. 22, No. 7, pp. (1269-1276)

Schnelle, M, Grotenhermen, F, Reif, M, Gorter, RW. (1999). [Results of a standardized survey on the medical use of cannabis products in the German-speaking area]. *Forsch Komplementarmed,* Vol. 6 Suppl 3, No. pp. (28-36)

Schon, F, Hart, PE, Hodgson, TL, Pambakian, AL, Ruprah, M, Williamson, EM, Kennard, C. (1999). Suppression of pendular nystagmus by smoking cannabis in a patient with multiple sclerosis. *Neurology,* Vol. 53, No. 9, pp. (2209-2210)

Scotter, E, Graham, S, Glass, M (2006) Cannabinoid Receptor Signal Transduction Pathways. In: *Cannabinoids: Structure and Function*, Reggio, P (ed): Humana Press.

Selvarajah, D, Gandhi, R, Emery, CJ, Tesfaye, S. (2010). Randomized placebo-controlled double-blind clinical trial of cannabis-based medicinal product (Sativex) in painful diabetic neuropathy: depression is a major confounding factor. *Diabetes Care,* Vol. 33, No. 1, pp. (128-130)

Skrabek, RQ, Galimova, L, Ethans, K, Perry, D. (2008). Nabilone for the treatment of pain in fibromyalgia. *J Pain,* Vol. 9, No. 2, pp. (164-173)

Smith, PF. (2004). GW-1000. GW Pharmaceuticals. *Curr Opin Investig Drugs.,* Vol. 5, No. 7, pp. (748-754)

Spector, M. (1973). Acute vestibular effects of marijuana. *J Clin Pharmacol,* Vol. 13, No. 5, pp. (214-217)

Stambaugh, JE, Jr., McAdams, J, Vreeland, F. (1984). Dose ranging evaluation of the antiemetic efficacy and toxicity of intramuscular levonantradol in cancer subjects with chemotherapy-induced emesis. *J Clin Pharmacol,* Vol. 24, No. 11-12, pp. (480-485)

Svendsen, KB, Jensen, TS, Bach, FW. (2004). Does the cannabinoid dronabinol reduce central pain in multiple sclerosis? Randomised double blind placebo controlled crossover trial. *Bmj,* Vol. 329, No. 7460, pp. (253)

Swift, W, Gates, P, Dillon, P. (2005). Survey of Australians using cannabis for medical purposes. *Harm Reduct J,* Vol. 2, No. pp. (18)

Valenzano, KJ, Tafesse, L, Lee, G, Harrison, JE, Boulet, JM, Gottshall, SL, Mark, L, Pearson, MS, Miller, W, Shan, S, Rabadi, L, Rotshteyn, Y, Chaffer, SM, Turchin, PI, Elsemore, DA, Toth, M, Koetzner, L, Whiteside, GT. (2005). Pharmacological and pharmacokinetic characterization of the cannabinoid receptor 2 agonist, GW405833, utilizing rodent models of acute and chronic pain, anxiety, ataxia and catalepsy. *Neuropharmacology.,* Vol. 48, No. 5, pp. (658-672)

van der Stelt, M, Di Marzo, V. (2005). Anandamide as an intracellular messenger regulating ion channel activity. *Prostaglandins Other Lipid Mediat,* Vol. 77, No. 1-4, pp. (111-122)

Van Sickle, MD, Duncan, M, Kingsley, PJ, Mouihate, A, Urbani, P, Mackie, K, Stella, N, Makriyannis, A, Piomelli, D, Davison, JS, Marnett, LJ, Di Marzo, V, Pittman, QJ, Patel, KD, Sharkey, KA. (2005). Identification and functional characterization of brainstem cannabinoid CB2 receptors. *Science,* Vol. 310, No. 5746, pp. (329-332)

Wade, DT, Makela, P, Robson, P, House, H, Bateman, C. (2004). Do cannabis-based medicinal extracts have general or specific effects on symptoms in multiple sclerosis? A double-blind, randomized, placebo-controlled study on 160 patients. *Mult Scler,* Vol. 10, No. 4, pp. (434-441)

Wade, DT, Makela, PM, House, H, Bateman, C, Robson, P. (2006). Long-term use of a cannabis-based medicine in the treatment of spasticity and other symptoms in multiple sclerosis. *Mult Scler,* Vol. 12, No. 5, pp. (639-645)

Wade, DT, Robson, P, House, H, Makela, P, Aram, J. (2003). A preliminary controlled study to determine whether whole-plant cannabis extracts can improve intractable neurogenic symptoms. *Clin Rehabil,* Vol. 17, No. 1, pp. (21-29)

Wallace, M, Schulteis, G, Atkinson, JH, Wolfson, T, Lazzaretto, D, Bentley, H, Gouaux, B, Abramson, I. (2007). Dose-dependent effects of smoked cannabis on capsaicin-induced pain and hyperalgesia in healthy volunteers. *Anesthesiology,* Vol. 107, No. 5, pp. (785-796)

Ware, MA, Adams, H, Guy, GW. (2005). The medicinal use of cannabis in the UK: results of a nationwide survey. *Int J Clin Pract,* Vol. 59, No. 3, pp. (291-295)

Ware, MA, Doyle, CR, Woods, R, Lynch, ME, Clark, AJ. (2003). Cannabis use for chronic non-cancer pain: results of a prospective survey. *Pain,* Vol. 102, No. 1-2, pp. (211-216)

Ware, MA, Gamsa, A, Persson, J, Fitzcharles, MA. (2002). Cannabis for chronic pain: case series and implications for clinicians. *Pain Res Manag,* Vol. 7, No. 2, pp. (95-99)

Watanabe, K, Yamaori, S, Funahashi, T, Kimura, T, Yamamoto, I. (2007). Cytochrome P450 enzymes involved in the metabolism of tetrahydrocannabinols and cannabinol by human hepatic microsomes. *Life Sci,* Vol. 80, No. 15, pp. (1415-1419)

Wissel, J, Haydn, T, Muller, J, Brenneis, C, Berger, T, Poewe, W, Schelosky, LD. (2006). Low dose treatment with the synthetic cannabinoid Nabilone significantly reduces spasticity-related pain : a double-blind placebo-controlled cross-over trial. *J Neurol,* Vol. 253, No. 10, pp. (1337-1341)

Wood, PB, Holman, AJ, Jones, KD. (2007). Novel pharmacotherapy for fibromyalgia. *Expert Opin Investig Drugs,* Vol. 16, No. 6, pp. (829-841)

Woolridge, E, Barton, S, Samuel, J, Osorio, J, Dougherty, A, Holdcroft, A. (2005). Cannabis use in HIV for pain and other medical symptoms. *J Pain Symptom Manage,* Vol. 29, No. 4, pp. (358-367)

Yu, XH, Cao, CQ, Martino, G, Puma, C, Morinville, A, St-Onge, S, Lessard, E, Perkins, MN, Laird, JM. (2010). A peripherally restricted cannabinoid receptor agonist produces robust anti-nociceptive effects in rodent models of inflammatory and neuropathic pain. *Pain,* Vol. 151, No. 2, pp. (337-344)

Zajicek, J, Fox, P, Sanders, H, Wright, D, Vickery, J, Nunn, A, Thompson, A. (2003). Cannabinoids for treatment of spasticity and other symptoms related to multiple sclerosis (CAMS study): multicentre randomised placebo-controlled trial. *Lancet,* Vol. 362, No. 9395, pp. (1517-1526)

Zajicek, JP, Sanders, HP, Wright, DE, Vickery, PJ, Ingram, WM, Reilly, SM, Nunn, AJ, Teare, LJ, Fox, PJ, Thompson, AJ. (2005). Cannabinoids in multiple sclerosis (CAMS) study: safety and efficacy data for 12 months follow up. *J Neurol Neurosurg Psychiatry,* Vol. 76, No. 12, pp. (1664-1669)

5

# Fibromyalgia Syndrome and Spa Therapy

Antonella Fioravanti[1], Nicola Giordano[2] and Mauro Galeazzi[1]
[1]*Rheumatology Unit, Department of Clinical Medicine and Immunological Sciences, The University of Siena*
[2]*Department of Internal Medicine, Endocrine and Metabolic Diseases, The University of Siena*
*Italy*

## 1. Introduction

Fibromyalgia syndrome (FS) is a common musculo-skeletal disorder characterized by otherwise unexplained chronic widespread pain, a lowered pain threshold, high tender point counts (tenderness on examination at specific, predictable anatomic sites known as tender points), sleep disturbances, fatigue, headache, irritable bowel syndrome, morning stiffness, paraesthesias in the extremities, often psychological distress and depressed mood (Mease, 2005).

The diagnosis of FS is based on a history of widespread pain, defined as bilateral, upper and lower body, as well as spine, and the presence of excessive tenderness on applying pressure to 11 of 18 specific muscle-tendon sites (Wolfe et al., 1990). The 1990 American College of Rheumatology (ACR) classification criteria for the diagnosis of FS provide a sensitivity and specificity of nearly 85% in differentiating FS from other forms of chronic musculoskeletal pain. According to these criteria, FS can be diagnosed in about 2-3% in the United States population, with a prevalence in women of 3.4% and in men of about 0.5% (Wolfe & Cathey, 1983). The most recent data from US describes FS as the third most prevalent rheumatic disease, after low back pain and osteoarthritis (Lawrence et al., 2008).

FS has a negative impact on quality of life (QoL), working capacity, family life and social functioning. Significantly higher total healthcare costs have been reported among patients diagnosed with FS compared to the general population (Spaeth, 2009); in fact, FS patients incur high direct medical costs and significant indirect costs (e.g. disability pension, absenteeism). Effective treatment options are therefore needed for medical and economic reasons.

Because of the unknown aetiology and the unclear pathogenesis, there is no standard therapy regime for FS. In recent years, at least three sets of guidelines have been developed by different medical organizations in an attempt to standardize the treatment of this condition (American Pain Society, European League Against Rheumatism, Association of the Medical Society of Germany) (Goldenberg et al., 2004 ; Carville et al., 2008 ; Klement et al., 2008). The current recommendations suggest that the optimal treatment of FS requires a multidisciplinary approach with a combination of non-pharmacological and pharmacological treatment modalities tailored according to pain intensity, function, associated features, such as depression, fatigue and sleep disturbances, decided through discussion with the patient. A variety of medical treatments, including antidepressants, opioids, analgesics, non-steroidal anti-inflammatory drugs (NSAIDs), sedatives, muscle relaxants and antiepileptics have been used to treat FS (Goldenberg et al., 2004 ; Carville et al., 2008 ; Klement et al., 2008). Given the complexity and chronicity of FS and the relatively poor response to pharmacological treatments, it is not surprising that patients often resort to complementary or alternative therapies (Sarac & Gur, 2006). Non-pharmaceutical treatment modalities, including exercise, physical therapy, massage, acupuncture, osteopathic manipulation, patient education and cognitive behavioural therapy can be helpful (Goldenberg et al., 2004 ; Carville et al., 2008 ; Klement et al., 2008). Spa therapy is one of the most commonly used non-pharmacological approaches for FS in many European countries, as well as in Japan and Israel. Spa therapy comprises a broad spectrum of therapeutic options including hydrotherapy, balneotherapy, physiotherapy, mud-pack therapy and exercise (Sukenik et al., 1999; Bender et al., 2005). However, despite their long history and popularity, spa treatments are still the subject of debate and their role in modern medicine is still not clear (Verhagen et al., 2000). We summarize the currently available information on clinical effects and mechanism of action of spa therapy in FS.

## 2. Randomized clinical trials (RCTs) on spa therapy in FS

We conducted a search of the literature in April 2011. In an attempt to standardize the patient sample included, the search was conducted from 1990 (the date of publication of the ACR classification criteria for FS) to April 2011. Medline was searched using the term "randomized clinical trial", "spa therapy", "mud" and "balneotherapy" in combination with FS. RCTs written in languages other than English were excluded from the search.

We identified eight assessable articles reporting 7 RCTs on spa therapy in FS, including a total number of patients of 314 (TABLE 1). Over 90% of the participants in the studies were women. All studies were blind with an "assessor" blind to the type of treatment. In five studies mineral baths were used, in one study bathing was combined with exercise treatment, one study evaluated the effect of spa therapy and one study the effect of mud-pack treatment.

Yurtkuran et al. (Yurtkuran et al., 1996) investigated the effect of the addition of balneotherapy to relaxation exercises in 40 patients with FS. The study was conducted in a daily living environment and the treatment duration was 2 weeks. Patients taking part in the balneotherapy program bathed at 37°C for 20 min a day, 5 days per week followed by relaxation exercises. Patients in the control group received only relaxation exercises. Pain relief, as scored by Visual Analogue Scale (VAS), was achieved in both groups at the end of therapy and persisted for 6 weeks; however, significant improvements in mean Pressure Algometric Scores (PAS) during follow-up were only observed in the balneotherapy group.

Buskila et al. (Buskila et al., 2001) and Neumann et al. (Neumann et al., 2001) reported the beneficial effect of Dead Sea balneotherapy on FS-related symptoms and QoL index in patients with FS. In this study 48 patients with FS were randomly assigned to treatment and control groups of 24 subjects each. The patients in the treatment group bathed for 20 min per day in a sulphur pool at 37°C for 10 days, while the control group did not receive this

| Authors | Sample size | Intervention | Outcome measures | Follow-up | Results |
|---|---|---|---|---|---|
| Yurtkuran 1996 | A: 20<br>B: 20 | A:Balneotherapy+ exercises<br>B:Excercises only | VAS, PAS | 6 weeks | Significant changes on VAS and PAS for group A at the end of treatment and at 6 weeks |
| Buskila 2001 | A: 24<br>B: 24 | A: Balneotherapy<br>B: No treatment | VAS (Pain and other minor symptoms), FIQ, TPC, Dolorimeter, FDI | 3 months | Significant between group improvements in pain and TPC in favour of A. Still seen after 3 months |
| Neumann 2001 | A: 24<br>B: 24 | A: Balneotherapy<br>B: No treatment | SF36, AIMS, VAS (Pain and other minor symptoms), | 3 months | Significant improvement in most subscales of the SF36 for both groups. The improvement in physical components of the QoL index lasted 3 months, whereas improvement in measures of psychological well-being was of shorter duration. Subjects in group A reported greater and longer-lasting improvement than subjects in the group B |
| Evcik 2002 | A: 22<br>B: 20 | A: Balneotherapy<br>B: No treatment | VAS, FIQ, TPC, BDI | 6 months | The group A showed statistically significant improvements in TPC, VAS, FIQ and BDI at the end of the therapy and this improvement persisted at 6 months except for BDI |
| Dönmez 2005 | A: 16<br>B: 14 | A :Spa therapy<br>B: No treatment | VAS (Pain and other minor symptoms), FIQ, TPC, BDI | 9 months | Significant improvements in pain, TPC and FIQ for group A. The pain and TPC results persisted for up to one month and the FIQ results for up to 6 months |
| Ardiç 2007 | A: 12<br>B: 12 | A: Balneotherapy<br>B: No treatment | VAS, TPC, FIQ, BDI | 3 weeks | Statistically significant improvement in VAS, BDI, TPC and FIQ was only found in group A at the end of the treatment cycle |
| Fioravanti 2007 | A: 40<br>B: 40 | A: Mud -packs and Baths<br>B: No treatment | FIQ, TPC, VAS (Pain and other minor symptoms), AIMS, HAQ | 16 weeks | In group A, a significant improvement in all parameters was recorded after mud-bath therapy and after 16 weeks |
| Özkurt 2011 | A: 25<br>B: 25 | A: Balneotherapy<br>B: No treatment | VAS, FIQ, BDI, PGA, IGA, SF-36, TPC | 3 months | Statistically significant improvement was recorded in group A for all outcome parameters at the end of the treatment cycle and after 3 months, except for BDI and IGA |

Table 1. RCTs on SPA Therapy in FS (1996-2011)

treatment. All participants stayed in the Dead Sea area for 10 days and continued their regular medications for FS. Physical functioning, assessed by the Fibromyalgia Impact Questionnaire (FIQ), FS-related symptoms, assessed by VAS, Functional Disability Index (FDI), Health Assessment Questionnaire (HAQ), tenderness measurements (Tender Point Count [TPC] and dolorimetry) and QoL index (Short Form-36 [SF36] and Arthritis Impact Measurement Scales [AIMS]) were recorded at basal time, at the end of treatment and 1 month and 3 months later. Physical functioning and tenderness improved moderately in both groups. With the exception of tenderness threshold, the improvement was especially evident in the treatment group and even persisted beyond 3 months. Relief in the severity of FS-related symptoms (pain, fatigue, stiffness) and reduced frequency of symptoms (headache, sleep problems and subjective joint swelling) were reported in both groups, but lasted longer in the treatment group. Significant improvement in most subscales of the SF36 was reported for both groups. Interestingly, the improvement in physical components of the QoL index usually lasted 3 months, whereas improvement in measures of psychological well-being was of shorter duration. Subjects in the balneotherapy group reported greater and longer-lasting improvement than subjects in the control group. Improvements in the control group were explained by temporary changes in lifestyle combined with the relaxed atmosphere of the Dead Sea resort.

Evcik et al. (Evcik et al., 2002) also reported significant improvements lasting up to 6 months in patients treated with balneotherapy. In this study 42 patients with FS were randomly assigned to two groups. One group (22 patients) bathed for 20 min at 36°C once a day, five times per week for 3 consecutive weeks (total 15 sessions) and the other group (20 patients) continued their regular medications without balneotherapy. Patients were evaluated by TPC, VAS for pain, Beck's Depression Index (BDI) and FIQ at basal time, after therapy and 6 months later. The balneotherapy group showed statistically significant improvements in TPC, VAS score, FIQ and BDI values at the end of therapy; at 6 months, the improvement in all parameters except BDI persisted.

A study by Donmez et al. (Donmez et al., 2005) compared the effects of a stay at a spa centre plus balneotherapy and the effects of regular care (control), recording significant improvements in major outcome measures, such as pain, TPC and FIQ with respect to control. The pain and TPC results persisted for up to one month and the FIQ results for up to 6 months. However, they could also be attributed to the effects of the spa stay (not offered to controls, who continued their habitual medical treatment and/or daily exercises).

Ardiç et al. (Ardiç et al., 2007) investigated the clinical effects of balneotherapy in the treatment of FS, considering serum levels of certain inflammatory markers. One group of patients (n=22) bathed 20 min per day for five days per week for three consecutive weeks and the other group (n=22) (control) continued with pharmacological treatment. A statistically significant improvement in algometric score, VAS, BDI, TPC and FIQ was only found in the balneotherapy group at the end of the treatment cycle.

In a multicentric single-blind RCT study, Fioravanti et al. (Fioravanti et al., 2007) assessed the effects of a combination of mud packs and thermal baths (with two types of mineral water) on patients with primary FS who responded poorly to pharmacological therapy. They also analysed tolerance to mud packs, since no trial using this thermal treatment has been performed in FS. Eighty patients with primary FS were randomly allocated to two groups: 40 underwent a cycle of 12 mud packs and thermal baths over a period of 2 weeks,

40 were enrolled as controls and continued their regular outpatient care routine. Because many other non-specific factors may also contribute to the effects observed after spa therapy, including changes in the environment, pleasant scenery and the absence of work duties, in order to temper these factors, all patients lived near the spa, continued working and did not modify their lifestyles. Another aspect that often amplifies the effects of spa therapy is its frequent association with physio-kinesiotherapy. These treatments were excluded from the protocol if they had not yet begun and were not already established. The following parameters were evaluated at baseline, after thermal treatment and after 16 weeks: FIQ, TPC, VAS for "minor" symptoms, AIMS1 and HAQ. Controls were assessed at the same intervals. A significant improvement in all parameters was recorded after mud-pack therapy and after 16 weeks.

Figure 1 shows that the patients submitted to mud-bath therapy underwent an evident improvement of VAS score at the end of the cycle of the thermal treatment cycle (T1) and this improvement remained significant after a follow-up period of 16 weeks (T2).

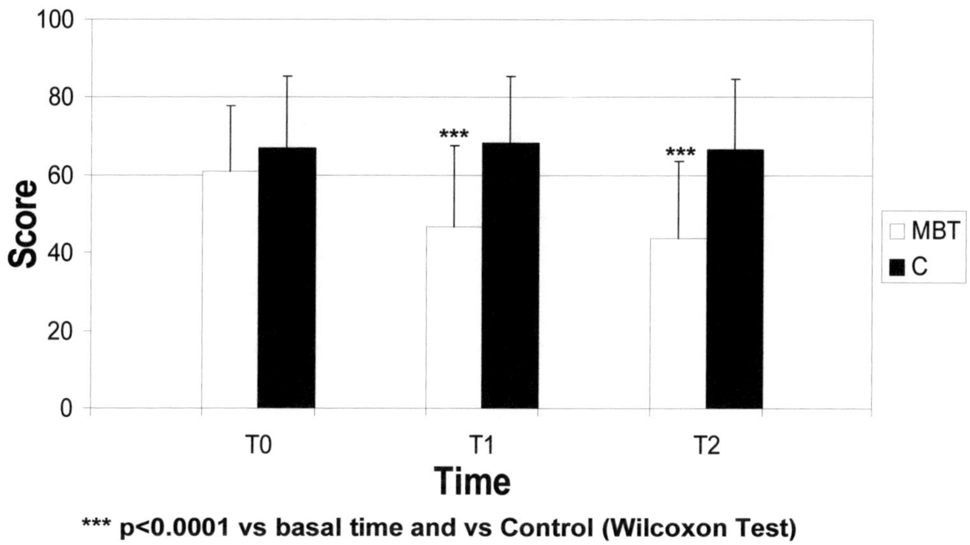


Fig. 1. VAS score (mean ± SD) at basal time (T0), after 2 weeks (T1) and 16 weeks (T2) in mud-bath treated patients (MBT) and in controls (C). From Fioravanti et al., Rheumatol Int 2007

Figure 2 demonstrates that TPC significantly was reduced at the end of the spa therapy cycle and remained stable after 16 weeks in comparison to baseline only in patients treated with mud-bath therapy.

The results were similar for the two types of mineral water. Regarding tolerance mud packs, no patient reported any exacerbation of symptoms and the hot applications were well tolerated by all. No drop-outs occurred during spa therapy and all patients completed the study.

A recent RCT by Özkurt et al. (Özkurt et al., 2011) of 50 woman with FS confirmed the efficacy of balneotherapy on major outcome measures such as pain, FIQ, BDI, Patient's and

Investigator's Global Assessment (PGA and IGA) scores, and SF36. The results were maintained for up to 3 months, except for BDI and investigator's global assessment score.

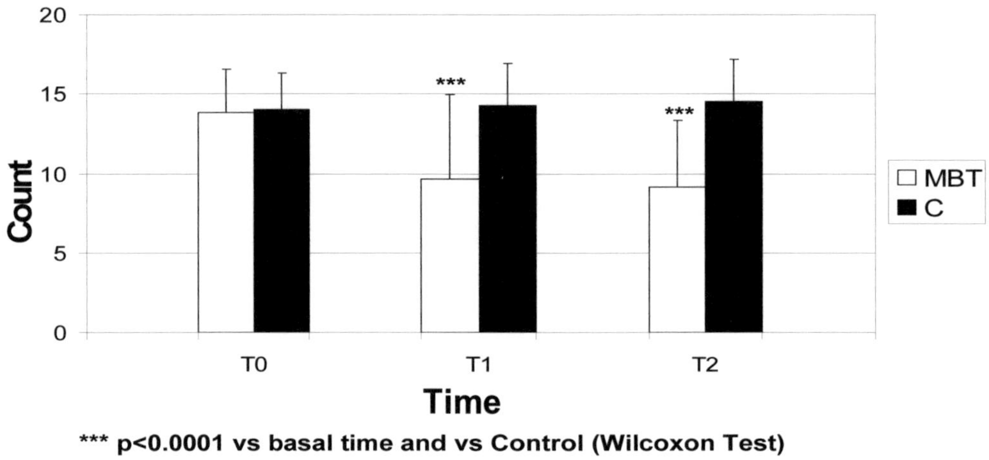


Fig. 2. Tender Point Count (mean ± SD) at basel time (T0), after 2 weeks (T1) and 16 weeks (T2) in mud-bath treated patients (MBT) and in controls (C). From Fioravanti et al. Rheumatol Int 2007

These various RCTs on spa therapy for FS suggest a positive effect on pain, other FS-related symptoms and QoL (McVeigh et al., 2008; Langhorst et al., 2009). The studies assessed the medium-long-term effect and found that the clinical efficacy of spa therapy lasted for 4-6 months. Despite low tolerance of physical treatments by FS patients, spa therapy seems to be well tolerated and to have a lower percentage of side effects, which are also less severe, than those associated with pharmacological treatments.

Some aspects of the studies on spa therapy for FS are disputable and could be a source of bias, for example the lack of double-blind experimental design due to the difficulty of creating a placebo with the same characteristics as the treatment. The methodological quality of the RCTs analysed was limited for the following reasons: 1) only two studies had a sample size of at least 25 per group, the number recognized as appropriate for detecting clinically significant differences between two active treatments (Chambless & Holton, 1998); 2) no study included intention-to-treat analysis, but analysed the completers, possibly favouring the results of spa therapy, even if the drop-out rates were low; 3) most studies did not report the method of randomization used; 4) the trials did not ensure that treatment allocation was concealed (McVeigh et al., 2008; Langhorst et al., 2009).

Comparison of the studies was difficult as the baseline characteristics of the patients were heterogeneous, the interventions differed in type, intensity and duration, the methods used for assessment of efficacy varied and patients were assessed at different times after spa therapy. In particular, the heterogeneity of "spa therapy" makes it difficult to determine which form of spa therapy is most effective and no study was designed to compare different types of spa care procedures.

Although the consistency of the results suggests that spa therapy has a therapeutic effect on FS, the methodological limitations of the studies preclude any definitive conclusions.

Studies conducted according to rigorous methodological criteria in larger numbers of patients are needed to determine the potential of spa therapy for FS.

### 2.1 Mechanisms of action of spa therapy in FS

The mechanisms by which immersion in mineral or thermal water or the application of mud alleviates suffering in FS are not fully understood. The net benefit is probably the result of a combination of factors, among which mechanical, thermal and chemical effects are most prominent (Sukenik et al., 1999; Fioravanti et al., 2011). A distinction can be made between the non-specific (hydrotherapeutic in a broad sense) mechanisms of simple bathing in hot tap water, and specific (hydromineral and crenotherapeutic) mechanisms, which depend on the chemical and physical properties of the water used. While the former are well known, the latter are difficult to identify and assess. Buoyancy, immersion, resistance and temperature all play important roles. Hot stimuli may influence muscle tone and pain intensity, helping to reduce muscle spasm and to increase the pain threshold in nerve endings. According to the "gate theory", pain relief may be due to the temperature and hydrostatic pressure of water on the skin (Melzack & Wall, 1965 ).

Thermal stress provokes a series of neuroendocrine reactions (Kuczera & Kokot, 1996), in particular release of adrenocorticotropic hormone (ACTH), cortisol, prolactin and growth hormone (GH), although it does not alter the circadian rhythm of these hormones. The effect of thermal stress on the hypothalamus-pituitary-adrenal axis seems to be particularly important for the antiedemigenous and anti-inflammatory effects of corticosteroids. Pituitary activation could also be particularly useful in FS, where altered reactivity of the hypothalamic-pituitary axis has been observed (Gur et al., 2004).

The increase in beta-endorphin demonstrated to occur with various spa therapy techniques has an analgesic and anti-spastic effect that is particularly important in patients with FS for whom pain is the prevalent symptom. Interestingly, it has been found that application of mature thermal mud in healthy individuals brings about a rapid increase in plasma beta-endorphin, which returns to pre-treatment levels within the period of the so-called thermal reaction (Cozzi et al., 1995). This increase in beta-endorphin is probably the key factor in the mechanism of individual tolerance to thermal mud baths. A recent study has shown a reduction in circulating levels of interleukin (IL)-1, prostaglandin E2 (PGE2) and leukotriene B4 (LTB4), important mediators of inflammation and pain, in FS patients undergoing a cycle of balneotherapy (Ardiç et al., 2007). It has been suggested that inflammatory process mediated by cytokines, proteases and inflammatory mediators located in soft body tissue may play a role in the pathogenesis of FS, in up to one third of FS patients (Salemi et al., 2003). This inflammatory process would stimulate subcutaneous nociceptors, resulting in a sensation of pain. The detection of IL-1, IL-6 and tumour necrosis factor-$\alpha$(TNF-$\alpha$) in skin of one-third of FS patients and elevated plasma PGE2 levels in FS supports this hypothesis (Hedenberg-Magnusson et al., 2001). The inhibitory effect of balneotherapy on the production and/or release of IL-1, PGE2 and LTB4 could explain the mechanism of clinical benefits of spa therapy in this disorder. Mineral water may also influence the oxidant-antioxidant system (Eckmekcioglu et al., 2002; Bender et al., 2007), which could be beneficial, since oxidative stress disorders have been described in FS (Bagis et al., 2005). Finally, other aspects of the mechanisms of mud packs and balneotherapy in FS need to be considered; for example, the climatic and environmental conditions of spas and the fact that people relax away from their daily routines (Sukenik et al., 1999; Fioravanti et al., 2011).

## 3. Conclusion

In conclusion, spa therapy seems to have a role in the treatment of FS. It cannot substitute for conventional therapy but can complement to it. The improvement reported in some clinical studies lasts over time. Actually, spa therapy can represent a useful backup to pharmacologic treatment of FS or a valid alternative for patients who do not tolerate pharmacologic treatments. Future research to clarify the mechanisms of action and the effects deriving from the application of thermal treatments are imperative. Additional RCTs with high methodological quality concerning the effectiveness of spa therapy in FS are necessary in order to obtained strong evidence on the effects of spa therapy.

## 4. References

Ardiç, F.; Őzgen, M.; Aybek, H.; Rota, S.; Cubukçu, D.; Gökgöz, A. (2007). Effects of balneotherapy on serum IL-1, PGE2 and LTB4 levels in fibromyalgia patients. *Rheumatology International,* Vol. 27, No. 5, (March), pp. 441-6, Print ISSN: 0172-8172 Online ISSN: 1437-160X

Bagis, S.; Tamer, L.; Sahin, G.; Bilgin, R.; Guler, H.; Ercan, B.; Erdogan, C.;(2005). Free radicals and antioxidants in primary fibromyalgia: an oxidative stress disorder?. *Rheumatology International,* Vol. 25, No. 3, (April), pp.188-90, Print ISSN: 0172-8172 Online ISSN: 1437-160X

Bender, T.; Karagülle, Z.; Bàlint, G.P.; Gutenbrunner, C.; Bàlint, P.V.; Sukenik, S. (2005). Hydrotherapy, balneotherapy, and spa treatment in pain management. *Rheumatology International,* Vol. 25, No. 3, (April), pp. 220-224, Print ISSN: 0172-8172 Online ISSN: 1437-160X

Bender, T.; Bariska, J.; Vàghy, R.; Gomez, R.; Kovàcs, I. (2007). Effect of balneotherapy on the Antoxidant System - A controlled pilot study. *Archives of Medical Research,* Vol.38, No.1, (January), pp. 86-89, ISSN: 0188-4409

Buskila, D.; Abu-Shakra, M.; Neumman, L.; Odes, L.; Shneider. E.; Flusser, D.; Sukenik, S. (2001). Balneotherapy for fibromyalgia at the Dead Sea. *Rheumatology International,* Vol. 20, No. 3, pp. 105-8, Print ISSN: 0172-8172 Online ISSN: 1437-160X

Carville, S.F.; Arendt-Nielsen, S.; Bliddal, H.; Blotman, F.; Branco, J.C. ;Buskila, D.; Da Silva, J.A.; Danneskiold-Samsøe, B.; Dincer, F.; Henriksson, C.; Henriksson, K.G.; Kosek, E.; Longley, K.; McCarthy, G.M.; Perrot, S.; Puszczewicz, M.; Sarzi-Puttini, P.; Silman, A.; Späth, M.; Choy, E.H. (2008). EULAR evidence- based recommendations for the management of fibromyalgia syndrome. *Annals of the Rheumatic Diseases,* Vol. 67, No.4, (April), pp. 536-541, Online ISSN 1468-2060

Chambless, D. & Holton, S. (1998). Defining empirically supported therapies. *Journal Consulting and Clinical Psychology,* Vol. 66, No. 1, (February), pp. 7-18, ISSN: 0022-006X

Cozzi, F.; Lazzarin, I.; Todesco, S.; Cima, L.; (1995). Hypotalamic pituary-adrenal axis dysregulation in healthy subjects undergoing mud-bath-applications. *Arthritis & Rheumatism,* Vol. 37, No. 8,(August), pp. 724-725, Online ISSN: 1529-0131

Dönmez, A.; Zeki Karagülle, M.; Tercan, N.; Dinler, M.; Işsever, H.; Karagülle, M.; Turan, M. (2005). SPA therapy in fibromyalgia: a randomised controlled clinic study. *Rheumatology International,* Vol. 26, No. 2, (December), pp. 168-72, Print ISSN: 0172-8172 Online ISSN: 1437-160X

Eckmekcioglu, C.; Strauss-Blasche, G.; Holzer, F.; Marktl, W. (2002). Effect of sulfur baths on antioxidative defense systems, peroxide concentrations and lipid levels in patients with degenerative osteoarthritis. *Forsch Komplementarmed Klass Naturheilkd,* Vol. 9, No. 4, (August), pp.216-20, Print ISSN: 1424-7364

Evcik, D.; Kizilay, B.; Gökçen, E. (2002). The effects of balneotherapy on fibromyalgia patients. *Rheumatology International,* Vol. 22, No. 2, (June), pp. 56-9, Print ISSN: 0172-8172 Online ISSN: 1437-160X

Fioravanti, A.; Perpignano, G.; Tirri, G.; Cardinale, G.; Gianniti, C.; Lanza, C.E.; Loi, A.; Tirri, E.; Sfriso, P.; Cozzi, F. (2007). Effects of mud-bath treatment on fibromyalgia patients: a randomized clinical trial. *Rheumatology International,* Vol. 27, No. 12, (October), pp. 1157-1161, Print ISSN: 0172-8172 Online ISSN: 1437-160X

Fioravanti, A.; Cantarini, L.; Guidelli, G.M.; Galeazzi, M. (2011). Mechanisms of action of spa therapies in rheumatic diseases: what scientific evidence is there? *Rheumatology International,* Vol. 31, No. 1, (January), pp. 1-8, Print ISSN: 0172-8172 Online ISSN: 1437-160X

Goldenberg, D.L.; Burckhardt, C.; Crofford, L. (2004). Management of fibromyalgia syndrome. *Journal of the American Medical Association,* Vol. 292, No. 19, (November), pp. 2388-2395, ISSN: 00987484

Gur, A.; Cevik, R.; Sarac, A.J.; Colpan, L.; Em, S. (2004). Hypothalamic-pituitary-gonadal axis and cortisol in young women with primary fibromyalgia: the potential roles of depression, fatigue, and sleep disturbance in the occurrence of hypocortisolism. *Annals of the Rheumatic Diseases,* Vol. 63, No. 11, (November), pp. 1504-1506, Online ISSN 1468-2060

Hedenberg-Magnusson, B.; Ernberg, M.; Alstergren, P.; Kopp S.; (2001). Pain mediation by prostaglandin E2 and leukotriene B4 in the human masseter muscle. *Acta Odontologica Scandinavica,* Vol. 59, No. 6, (December), pp. 348-55, Print ISSN: 0001-6357 Online 1502-3850

Klement, A.; Hauser, W.; Bruckle, W.; Eidmann, U.; Felde, E.; Herrmann, M.; Kühn-Becker, H.; Offenbächer, M.; Settan, M.; Schiltenwolf, M.; von Wachter, M.; Eich, W. (2008). Principles of treatment, coordination of medical care and patient education in fibromyalgia syndrome and chronic widespread pain. *Der Schmerz,* Vol. 22, No. 3, (June), pp. 283-294, ISSN: 1432-2129

Kuczera, M. & Kokot, F. (1996). The influence of SPA therapy on endocrine system. Stress reaction hormones. *Polskie Archiwum Medycyny Wewnętrznej,* Vol. 95, No. 1, (January), pp. 11-20, Print ISSN: 0032-3772 Online ISSN: 1897-9483

Langhorst, J.; Musial, F.; Klose, P.; Häuser, W. (2009). Efficacy of hydrotherapy in fibromyalgia syndrome-a meta-analysis of randomized controlled clinical trials. *Rheumatology,* Vol. 48, No. 9, (September), pp. 1155-1159, Print ISSN 1462-0324 Online ISSN 1462-0332

Lawrence, R.C.; Felson, D.T.; Helmick, C.G.; Arnold, L.M.; Choi, H.; Deyo, R.A.; Gabriel, S.; Hirsch, R.; Hochberg, M.C.; Hunder, G.G.; Jordan, J.M.; Katz, J.N.; Kremers, H.M.; Wolfe, F. (2008). Estimates of the prevalence of arthritis and other rheumatic conditions in the United States. Part II. *Arthritis & Rheumatism,* Vol. 58, No. 2, (January), pp. 26-35, Online ISSN: 1529-0131

Mease, P. (2005). Fibromyalgia syndrome: review of clinical presentation, pathogenesis, outcome measures and treatment. *The Journal of Rheumatology,* Vol. Suppl, No. 75, (August), pp. 6-21, Print ISSN: 0315-162X Online ISSN: 1499-2752

McVeigh, J.G.; McGaughey, H.; Hall, M.; Kane, P. (2008). The effectiveness of hydrotherapy in the management of fibromyalgia syndrome: a systematic review. *Rheumatology International,* Vol. 29, No. 2, (December), pp. 119-130, Print ISSN: 0172-8172 Online ISSN: 1437-160X

Melzack, R. & Wall, P.D. (1965). Pain mechanism: a new theory. *Science,* Vol. 150, No. 699, (November), pp. 971-979, Print ISSN: 0036-8075 Online ISSN: 1095-9203

Neumman, L.; Sukenik, S.; Bolotin, A.; Abu-Shakra, M.; Amir, M.; Flusser, D.; Buskila, D. (2001). The effect of balneotherapy at the Dead Sea on the quality of life of patients with fibromyalgia syndrome. *Clinical Rheumatology,* Vol. 20, No. 1, pp. 15-9, Print ISSN: 0770-3198 Online ISSN: 1434-9949

Ozkurt, S.; Dönmez, A.; Zeki Karagülle, M.; Uzunoglu, E.; Turan, M.; Erdogan, N. (2011). Balneotherapy in fibromyalgia: a single blind randomized controlled clinical study. *Rheumatology International,* (in press), Print ISSN: 0172-8172 Online ISSN: 1437-160X

Salemi, S.; Rethage, J.; Wollina, U.; Michel, B.A.; Gay, R.E.; Gay, S.; Sprott, H.; (2003). Detection of interleukin 1 beta (IL-1 beta), IL-6, and tumor necrosis factor-alpha in skin of patient with fibromyalgia. *The Journal of Rheumatology* , Vol. 30, No. 1, (January), pp. 146-50, Print ISSN: 0315-162X Online ISSN: 1499-2752

Sarac, A.J. & Gur, A. (2006). Complementary and alternative medical therapies in fibromyalgia. *Current Pharmaceutical Design,* Vol. 12, No. 1, pp. 47–57, Print ISSN: 1381-6128 Online ISSN:1873-4286

Spaeth, M. (2009). Epidemiology, costs, and the economic burden of fibromyalgia. *Arthritis Research Therapy,* Vol. 11, No. 3, (June), pp. 117, ISSN: 1478-6354

Sukenik, S.; Flusser, D.; Abu-Shakra, M. (1999). The role of SPA therapy in various rheumatic diseases. *Rheumatic Diseases Clinics of North America,* Vol. 25, No. 4, (November), pp. 883-897, Print ISSN: 0889-857X Online ISSN: 1558-316

Verhagen, A.P.; de Vet, H.C.; de Bie, R.A.; Kessels, A.G.; Boers, M.; Knipschild, P.G. (2000). Balneotherapy for rheumatoid arthritis and osteoarthritis. *Cochrane Database Syst Rev* 2:CD000518

Wolfe, F. & Cathey, M.A. (1983). Prevalence of primary and secondary fibrositis. *The Journal of Rheumatology,* Vol. 10, No. 6, (December), pp. 965-968, Print ISSN: 0315-162X Online ISSN: 1499-2752

Wolfe, F.; Smythe, H.A.; Yunus, M.B.; Bennett, R.M.; Bombardier, C.; Goldenberg, D.L.; Tugwell, P.; Campbell, S.M.; Abeles, M.; Clark, P. (1990). The American College of Rheumatology 1990 criteria for the classification of fibromyalgia. *Arthritis & Rheumatism,* Vol. 33, No 2, (February), pp. 160-72, Online ISSN: 1529-0131

Yurtkuran, M. & Celiktas, M. (1996). A randomized, controlled trial of balneotherapy in the treatment of patients with primary fibromyalgia syndrome. *Physical Medicine Rehabilitation Kuror,* Vol. 6,pp. 109-112, ISSN 09406689

# 6

# Efficacy of Spinal Cord Stimulation for Central Post-Stroke Pain

Mohamed Ali[1] and Youichi Saitoh[2,3]
*[1]Department of Neurosurgery, Mansura University*
*[2]Department of Neurosurgery, Osaka University Graduate School of Medicine*
*[3]Department of Neuromodulation and Neurosurgery, Osaka University,Osaka*
*[1]Egypt*
*[2,3]Japan*

## 1. Introduction

Central post-stroke pain (CPSP) is a neuropathic-type of pain that affects about 1-8% of patients after stroke (Andersen et al., 1995; Bowsher 1993), and is characterized by pain and sensory dysfunction involving the area of the body that has been affected by the stroke (Leijon et al., 1998). Once present, CPSP rarely abates, causing a considerable long-term impact on patient's quality of life (Wider & Ahlstrom, 2002). The first line of treatment for CPSP is usually tricyclic antidepressant amitriptyline or antiepileptic gabapentine. However, these drugs are often ineffective or cause intolerable side effects; including dry mouth, urinary retention, arrhythmias, and sedation; especially in elderly stroke patients (Finnerup et al., 2005).

Neuromodulatory techniques have been proposed for treatment of severe medically refractory CPSP (Kim, 2009). Deep brain stimulation (DBS) has yielded inconsistent results (Kumar et al., 1997). Motor cortex stimulation (MCS) has been the most popular technique to treat intractable CPSP. MCS involves implanting electrodes over the motor strip through a craniotomy. MCS has been reported to achieve pain relief in approximately half of patients (Katayama et al., 1998; Fontaine et al., 2009; Saitoh et al., 2007; Lazortheset al., 2006). However, a large proportion of patients remain untreated due to either failure or decline of MCS (Aly et al., 2010). One group of patients declined MCS because of the need for a craniotomy (Aly et al., 2010). Another group of patients are considered poor candidates for MCS based on their poor response to repeated transcranial Magnetic Stimulation (r TMS) (Hosomi et al., 2008; Andre-Obadia et al., 2006). Moreover, MCS needs a special neurosurgical expertise and its use is correspondingly restricted to well-established functional neurosurgical centers (Kim, 2009). In these situations, there is practically no viable option to help these patients to relive their disabling medically refractory pain (Aly et al., 2010).

Spinal cord stimulation (SCS) is the most widely used neurostimulation technique for chronic pain because it is minimally invasive, has a low complication rate, and is generally effective (Kumar et al., 2006; Camerons, 2004). SCS has been proven effective for various types of neuropathic pain of peripheral origin, in particular, failed back surgery syndrome (FBSS) and peripheral neuropathy (Kumar et al., 2006). In contrast, only a few reports to date have investigated the use of SCS for CPSP (Simpson, 1991; Katayama et al, 2001; Cruccu et al., 2007; Lopez al., 2009; Aly et al., 2010) . SCS is generally considered ineffective for central neuropathic pain, including CPSP in spite of the paucity of data in the literature to support this idea (Simpson, 1991; Katayama et al., 2001; Cruccu et al., 2007; Lopez et al., 2009; Aly et al., 2010). CPSP most often has a wide pain distribution and commonly occurs in a hemibody fashion (Kim, 2009). Because coverage of the entire painful area by stimulation paraesthesia is essential for success of SCS (Holsheimer, 1997), SCS was considered unsuitable for CPSP. From a pthophysiological point of view, it was argued how SCS which act on segmental spinal level would affect pain generators in CPSP which are located proximal to deafferentiation level i.e. supraspinal (Tsubokawa, et al., 1993).

In this chapter, we reviewed that literature about the use of SCS for CPSP with regard to patient selection, surgical technique, clinical outcome and, and mechanism of action.

## 2. Presurgical evaluation

The diagnosis of CPSP should be established based on the following criteria (Klit et al., 2009): 1) development of pain following stroke; 2) sensory disturbance correlated with the cerebrovascular lesion; 3) pain located within the territory of sensory disturbance. Other causes of nociceptive and peripheral neuropathic pain should be ruled out particularly those which are prevalent in this age group such as lumbar canal stenosis, peripheral neuropathy, and post-stroke shoulder pain (Kim, 2009; Aly et al., 2010).

Comprehensive neuropsychological assessment is essential in all patients to rule out serious psychiatric disorder or severe cognitive dysfunction (Kumar et al., 2006). To be eligible for SCS treatment, patients should have failed medical treatment for at least 6 months, including antidepressants and anticonvulsant drugs (Cruccu et al., 2007).

## 3. Patients selection for SCS

There is no doubt that MCS remains the primary option for treating intractable CPSP based upon the available literature (Fontaine et al., 2009; Saitoh et al., 2007; et al., 2008). The experience with MCS is larger and the outcome is more consistent. MCS hss been implanted in more than 117 patients with CPSP with approximately 50 % success rate (Fontaine et al., 2009). However, a significant proportion of patients with intractable CPSP remain untreated either due to failure, poor prediction, or refusal of MCS by patients. In a recent study, out of 87 patients presented to neurosurgery department with intractable CPSP only 13 patients eventually had underwent MCS (Aly et al., 2010).Therefore, SCS may be an alternative option in the following situations;

### 3.1 Failure or poor predictors of MCS

Approximately 50 % of patients who undergo MCS fail to have satisfactory pain relief (Fontaine et al., 2009; Saitoh et al., 2007; Hosomi et al., 2008). Another group of patients may be considered poor candidates for MCS based on their poor response to TMS (Saitoh et al., 2007; Hosomi et al., 2008; Aly et al., 2010). For those groups of patients SCS may be one of the few viable options.

### 3.2 Patient preference

Some patients may prefer SCS over MCS because it does not need of craniotomy or general anesthesia as MCS does (Aly al., 2010). Compared to MCS, percutaneous trial SCS is much better tolerated by patients can be done under local anesthesia, and the electrodes can be removed easily if a trial fails (Aly et al., 2010). In fact, the minimal invasiveness and simplicity of SCS is one of the most appealing aspects of SCS for clinicians and patients as well.

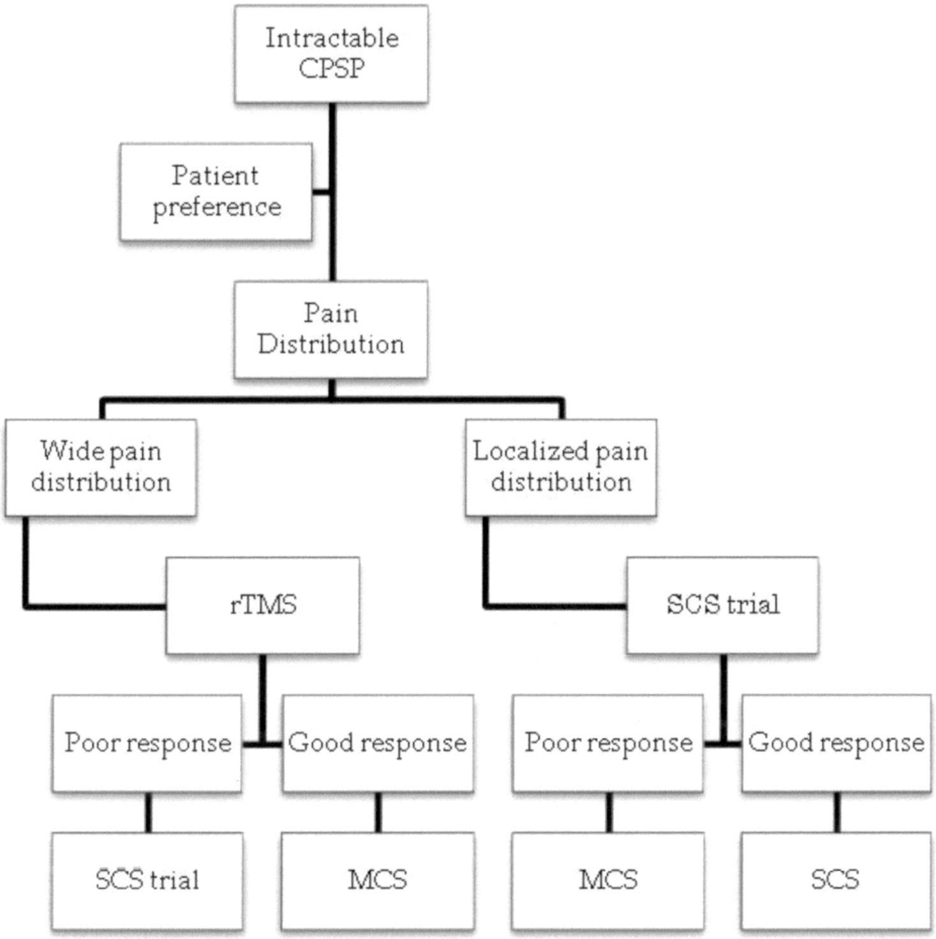


Fig. 1. Suggested algorithm for management of intractable CPSP.

### 3.3 Unavailability of MCS service

MCS service is generally less accessible than SCS. Because MCS needs a craniotomy and special neurosurgical expertise its use is limited to specialized neurosurgical centers (Aly et al., 2010). In contrast, the SCS technique is relatively simple, less invasive, and can be mastered not only by neurosurgeons but by many anesthesiologists and pain clinicians as well (Kim, 2009; Aly et al., 2010).

### 3.4 Pain distribution

#### 3.4.1 Localized pain distribution

The distribution of CPSP throughout the body may be quite variable. CPSP most often occurs in a hemibody fashion, but may be restricted to distal parts of the body, such as the hand or foot (Kim, 2009).Because coverage of the entire targeted region of pain by stimulation-induced paraesthesia is essential for success of SCS (Holsheimer, 1997), it was thought that SCS may be unsuitable for CPSP. Obviously, patients who have localized pain may be the ideal candidate for SCS. Patients with putaminal hemorrhage that affects the posterior part of the internal capsule has the propensity to cause pain that is most severe in, or confined to, the leg (Kim, 2003). This explains why that group of patients represented (40%) of cases in Ali et al study (Aly et al., 2010). Some patients have a wide pain distribution but pain is more severe in distal parts such as foot or hand which cause substantial disability due to interfering with hand movement or walking respectively (Aly et al., 2010). It was reported that targeting these distal areas which are most painful may still improve the patient pain. In this context it is helpful to measure a separate VAS rating of different areas. Finally, some patients will benefit from insertion of 2 different electrodes in cervical and dorsal spine to target a wide area (Aly et al., 2010).

#### 3.4.2 Lower extremity pain

Patients with leg-dominant CPSP were considered more suitable candidates for SCS than upper extremity pain because thoracic electrodes are technically less demanding and less susceptible to displacement than cervical electrodes. (Kumar & Wilson, 2007 ).In addition, lower-limb pain is not considered a good indication for MCS, given the technical difficulties associated with implanting electrodes on the medial surface of the brain (Fontaine et al., 2009;Aly et al., 2010).

## 4. Surgical procedure

### 4.1 Implantation of temporary electrodes

In the prone position, a percutaneous lead with quadripolar electrodes (Pisces Quad, Model 3487A; Medtronic, Inc., MN, USA) is inserted into the epidural space through a Touhy needle under local anesthesia. The tip was advanced to the required spinal level: C4 to C7 for upper limb pain or T9 to T12 for lower limb pain. The electrodes were manipulated with fluoroscopic guidance so that the stimulation-induced paraesthesia covered the entire region affected by pain (Aly et al., 2010; Stojanovic &Abdi, 2002; Kumar et al., 2006).

### 4.2 Trial stimulation

Using an externalized temporary lead connected to a test stimulator (model 3625, Medtronic), trial stimulation was performed to evaluate the efficacy of pain relief before permanent implantation. During the trial period (2 to 14 days), patients were allowed to test the pain-relieving effects of several stimulation parameters and combinations of active electrodes. Thereafter, the temporary electrodes are removed and patients were discharged. After counseling the patients in outpatient clinic, those who decided to proceed were scheduled for implantation of a permanent SCS system (Aly et al., 2010; Stojanovic & Abdi , 2002; Kumar , et al., 2006).

### 4.3 Implantation of permanent SCS system

A permanent lead was implanted in a similar manner as the trial lead and was anchored subcutaneously. Finally, an implantable pulse generator (IPG; Itrel III Model 7425 or Synergy Model 7427 V, Medtronic, Inc.) is implanted under general anesthesia in the left lower abdomen or anterior chest (Aly et al., 2010).

### 4.4 Evaluation of pain relief

Pain intensity was evaluated using a visual analogue scale (VAS) ranging from 0 (no pain) to 10 (worst possible pain) at baseline, during the trial, and at follow-up visits every 6 months. In patients with wide regions of pain, the VAS was assessed independently for each region and the target area for SCS was determined based on the area with greatest pain and disability(Aly MM, et al, 2010) (Fig. 2).

In addition, the patient global impression of change (PGIC) scale was assessed at the latest follow-up visit after the permanent implant. The PGIC scale indicates overall improvement according to a seven-point categorical scale: 1, very much improved; 2, much improved; 3, minimally improved; 4, no change; 5, minimally worse; 6, much worse; and 7, very much worse. The "rank 2" and "rank 1" were considered as clinically significant improvement (Aly MM, et al, 2010; Farrar, J., 2001).

During data analysis, the degree of pain relief was classified into three categories: good (≥50%), fair (30-49%), or poor (<30%) based on percent reduction of VAS (% reduction = [VAS pre-stimulation - VAS post-stimulation / VAS pre-stimulation] × 100%).13 Pain relief of "fair" or better was considered clinically significant based on a report documenting that pain reduction as low as 30 % corresponds to clinically meaningful success(Aly et al., 2010; Farrar,2001).

### 4.5 Stimulation parameters

The most common stimulation parameters were an amplitude of 1.5-3 V (range 1.5-6 V), a pulse width of 210 μsec (range 210-350 μsec), and a frequency of 31 Hz (range 10-50 Hz) with a bipolar configuration (Aly et al., 2010)

## 5. Clinical outcome

### 5.1 Previous studies design

To our knowledge, only 4 previous studies have investigated the use of SCS in CPSP (Table 1) (Simpson, 1991; Katayama, et al., 2001; Cruccu, et al., 2007; Lopez, 2009; Aly et al., 2010).

All previous studied were retrospective in nature and involved a small Number of patients (6-45). Therefore, a prospective controlled study with a larger population of patients is needed to provide stronger evidence for the efficacy of SCS in CPSP. However performing such study poses certain challenges. Firstly, it is difficult to recruit a large number of CPSP patients in one center owing to the low prevalence and under-diagnosis of this condition

(Kim, 2009).It is also difficult to conduct a placebo-controlled studies or blinded evaluations because SCS induces perceptible sensation (Camerons, 2004). Therefore, the role of placebo effect remains unresolved problem in SCS literature. Finally it is difficult to conduct case-matched controls, as in surgical practice long-term follow-up care is available only for surgically treated patients (Aly et al., 2010).

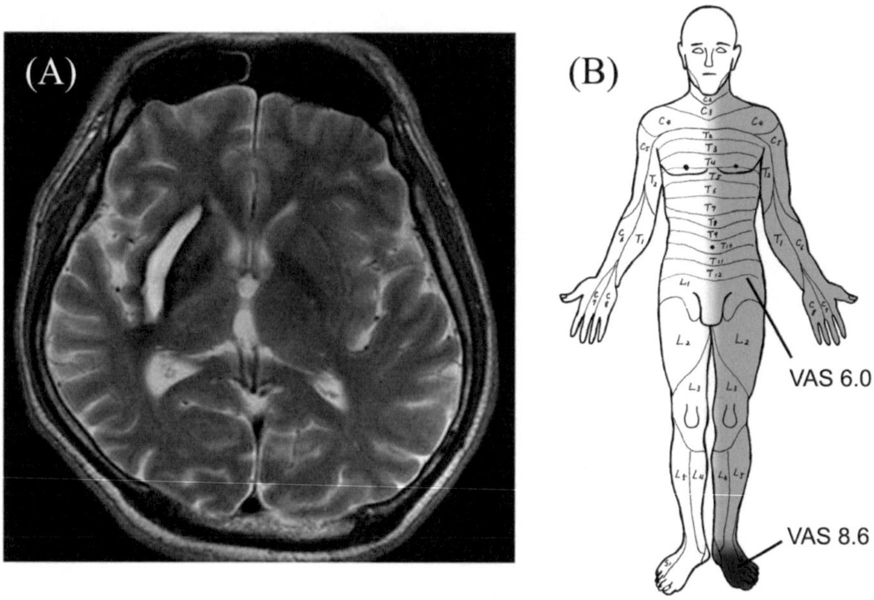


Fig. 2. MRI reveals evidence of an old right putaminal hemorrhage (A). The distribution of pain in the left hemibody shows that pain was more severe in the left foot; the patient therefore underwent implantation of a lower thoracic electrode targeting the foot region (B).

### 5.2 Success rate

Simpson et al first reported about long-term efficacy of SCS for CPSP in 10 patients (Simpson, 1991). Three out of the 10 patients (30 %) reported clinically significant improvement. The study done by Katayama was the main study reporting poor outcome from SCS (Katayama, et al, 2001) . Katayama reported long-term pain reduction (≥60%) in

| Authors | No of cases | Outcome measure | Pain distribution | Success rate % |
|---|---|---|---|---|
| Simpson, 1991 | 10 | Subjective improvement | Not available | 30 |
| Katayama, 2001 | 45 | VAS > 60 % | Not available | 7 |
| Ali, 2010 | 30 | VAS > 30 %,PGIC | Localized pain | 25 |
| Lopez, 2009 | 6 | VAS > 50 % | Localized pain | 80 |

Table 1. Summery of clinical outcomes of SCS studies for CPSP

only 3 of 45 patients (7%). Aly et al reported about 30 patients who underwent a trial of spinal cord stimulation, 10 underwent permanent placement, and 9 were available for follow-up (Aly, et al., 2010). Good or fair pain relief was seen in 7 of 9 patients (78%) with just over a mean 2-year follow-up. Lopez et al reported about 6 patients with SCS for CPSP. Good-to-excellent results were attained in 5 on long-term follow up (Lopez, et al., 2009).

### 5.3 Interpretation of outcome of previous studies

Three out of the 4 previous studies reported moderate to high success rate of SCS for CPSP (25-80 %). The fourth study reported a poor outcome from SCS with success rate of only 7 %.On interpreting the results of these studies it should be noted that these studies used different outcome measures and different inclusion criteria with regard to pain distribution (Table 1). Actually there is no consensus regarding what constitutes an optimum threshold for success in chronic pain studies. Most studies use the criterion of 50% pain relief as threshold of success. However, this criterion is increasingly challenged, because in clinical practice, patients will often be satisfied with 30% pain relief (Farrar et al., 2001; Cruccu et al., 2007). We therefore suspect that the use of > 60% VAS reduction by Katayama group might be unsuitably high threshold for success which may underestimated the clinical effect of SCS in this study (Aly et al, 2010).

### 5.4 Complications

Generally, the reported complication rate is low. Minor, clinically insignificant migrations were seen in 2 patients in one study (Aly et al., 2010). One electrode fractured and was replaced in another study (Lopez et al., 2009).

### 5.5 Predictors of success of SCS

Only one study analyzed the clinical factors predictive of success of SCS for CPSP (Aly et al., 2010).It was found that patients with hyperpathia tended to respond less well to trial stimulation than those without. This observation is consistent with a previous report in which SCS was less effective for control of evoked pain than spontaneous pain (Kim et al, 2001). It was also found that the effects of trial stimulation were sustained following permanent implantation in the majority of patients. SCS trial stimulation is thus advantageous for predicting efficacy in a minimally invasive manner before permanent implantation.

## 6. Mechanisms of action

The mechanism behind pain relieving effect of SCS is still not fully understood. Inhibition at spinal segmental level and activation of supraspinal mechanisms have been suggested as possible neurophysiologic mechanisms (Kishima et al., 2010). Positron emission tomography (PET) and functional magnetic resonance imaging (fMRI) studies had detected brain activation during SCS (Stancák et al., 2008). Using H215O PET, we have recently observed activation not only in somatosensory areas but also in those areas concerned with emotional aspects of pain such as anterior cingulate cortex and prefrontal areas (Kishima et al., 2010). CPSP is thought to be due to abnormal processing of nociceptive information rostral to the level of deaffrentiation (Katayama et al., 2001).

Therefore, we speculate that the pain relieving effect of SCS in CPSP may be interpreted in light of its supraspinal mechanisms (Aly et al., 2010)

## 7. Conclusion

SCS may provide improved pain control in a group of patients with medically intractable CPSP. The efficacy of SCS in CPSP is generally modest; both in terms of success rate and degree of pain relief. However, this modest degree of efficacy is important considering the severity of pain in these patients, the refractory nature of their pain, and the paucity of alterative therapeutic options. A further prospective controlled study with larger population of patients is still needed to provide stronger evidence for the efficacy of SCS in CPSP and define patient population who are most likely to get benefit from SCS treatment. SCS should be one of the neurostimulation techniques available to treat the medically-refractory post-stroke pain patient.

## 8. References

Andersen, G., Vestergaard, K., Ingeman-Nielsen, M., Jensen, T.S. (1995). Incidence of central post stroke pain. *Pain*, 61, 187-194.

Andre-Obadia, N., Peyron, R., Mertens, P., Mauguiere, F., Laurent, B., Garcia-Larrea, L. (2006). Transcranial magnetic stimulation for pain control. Double-blind study of different frequencies against placebo, and correlation with motor cortex stimulation efficacy. *Clin Neurophysiol*, 117, 1536-1544, ISSN 1388-2457

Bowsher, D. (1993). Cerebrovascular disease: Sensory consequences of stroke. Lancet, 341, 156.

Canavero, S., Bonicalzi, V. (2003). Spinal cord stimulation for central pain (Letter to Editor). *Pain*, 103, 228–228.719.

Cruccu, G., Aziz, T.Z., Garcia-Larrea, L., Hansson, P., Jensen, T.S., Lefaucheur, J.P., Simpson, B.A., Taylor, R.S. (2007). EFNS guidelines on neurostimulation therapy for neuropathic pain. *Eur J Neurol*, 14, 952-970.

Farrar, J.T., Young, J.P., LaMoreaux, L., Werth, J.L., Poole, R.M. (2001). Clinical importance of change in chronic pain intensity measured on an 11-point numerical pain rating scale. *Pain*, 94, 149-158.

Finnerup, N.B., Otto, M., McQuay, H.J., Jensen, T.S., Sindrup, S.H. (2005). Algorithm for neuropathic pain treatment: an evidence based proposal. *Pain*, 118, 289-305.

Fontaine, D., Hamani, C., and Lozano, A. (2009). Efficacy and safety of motor cortex stimulation for chronic neuropathic pain: critical review of the literature. *J Neurosurg*, 110, 251-256.

Holsheimer, J. (1997). Effectiveness of spinal cord stimulation in the management of chronic pain: analysis of technical drawbacks and solutions. *Neurosurgery*, 40, 990-996.

Hosomi, K., Saitoh, Y., Kishima, H., Oshino, S., Hirata, M., Tani, N., Shimokawa, T., Yoshimine, T. (2008). Electrical stimulation of primary motor cortex within the central sulcus for intractable neuropathic pain. *Clin Neurophysiol*, 119, 993-1001.

Katayama, Y., Fukaya, C., Yamamoto, T. (1998). Poststroke pain control by chronic motor cortex stimulation: neurological characteristics predicting a favorable response. *J Neurosurg*, 89, 585-91.

Katayama, Y., Yamamoto, T., Kobayashi, K., Kasai, M., Oshima, H., Fukaya, C. (2001). Motor cortex stimulation for post-stroke pain: comparison of spinal cord and thalamic stimulation. *Stereotaact Funct Neurosurg*, 77, 183-186.

Kim, J.S. (2003). Post-stroke central pain or paraesthesia after lenticulocapsular hemorrhage. Neurology, 61, 679-682.

Kim, J.S. (2009). Post-stroke pain. *Expert Rev Neurother*, 9, 711-721.

Kim, S.H., Tasker, R.R., Oh, M.Y. (2001). Spinal cord stimulation for nonspecific limb pain versus neuropathic pain and spontaneous versus evoked pain. *Neurosurgery*, 48, 1056-1064.

Kishima, H., Saitoh, Y., Oshino, S., Hosomi, K., Ali, M., Maruo, T., Hirata, M., Goto, T., Yanagisawa, T., Sumitani, M., Osaki, Y., Hatazawa, J., Yoshimine, T. (2010). Modulation of neuronal activity after spinal cord stimulation for neuropathic pain; H215O PET study. *Neuroimage*, 49, 2564-2569.

Klit, H., Finnerup, N.B., and Jensen, T.S. (2009). Central post-stroke pain: clinical characteristics, pathophysiology, and management. *Lancet Neurology*. 8, 857-868.

Kumar, K., Toth, C., Nath, R.K. (1997). Deep brain stimulation for intractable pain: a 15-year experience. *Neurosurgery* 1997;40:736–746.

Kumar, K., Hunter, G., Demeria, D. (2006). Spinal cord stimulation in treatment of chronic benign pain: challenges in treatment planning and present status, a 22-year experience. *Neurosurgery*, 58, 481-496.

Kumar, K., Wilson, J.R. (2007). Factors affecting spinal cord stimulation outcome in chronic benign pain with suggestions to improve success rate. *Acta Neurochir Suppl*, 97, 91-99.

Lazorthes, Y., Sol, J.C., Fowo, S., Roux, F.E., Verdie, J.C. (2007). Motor cortex stimulation for neuropathic pain. *Acta Neurochir*, 97 (Pt 2), 37–44.

Leijon, G., Boivie, J., and Johansson, I. (1989). Central post-stroke pain -neurological symptoms and pain characteristics. *Pain*, 36, 13-25.

Lopez, J.A., Torres, L.M., Gala, F., Iglesias, I. (2009). Spinal Cord Stimulation and Thalamic Pain: Long-term Results of Eight Cases. *Neuromodulation*, 12, 240-243.

Saitoh, Y., Yoshimine, T. (2007). Stimulation of primary motor cortex for intractable deafferentation pain. In: Sakas, D.E., Simpson, B.A., editors. *Operative neuromodulation, Vol. 2. Wein: Springer*, 51-6.

Saitoh, Y., Hirayama, A., Kishima, H., Shimokawa, T., Oshino, S., Hirata, M., Tani, N., Kato, A., Yoshimine, T. (2007). Reduction of intractable deafferentation pain due to spinal cord or peripheral lesion by high-frequency repetitive transcranial magnetic stimulation of the primary motor cortex. *J Neurosurg*, 107, 555-9.

Simpson, B.A. (1991). Spinal cord stimulation in 60 cases of intractable pain. *Journal of Neurol Neurosurg Psychiatry*, 54, 196-199.

Stancák, A., Kozák, J., Vrba, I., Tintera, J., Vrána, J., Polácek, H., Stancák, M. (2008). Functional magnetic resonance imaging of cerebral activation during spinal cord stimulation in failed back surgery syndrome patients. *Eur J Pain*, 12, 137-148.

Stojanovic, M., Abdi, S. (2002). Spinal Cord Stimulation. *Pain Phys.*, 5, 156-166.

Tracy, Camerons. (2004). Safety and efficacy of spinal cord stimulation for the treatment of chronic pain: a 20-year literature review. *J Neurosurg*, 100, 254-267.

Tsubokawa, T., Katayama, Y., Yamamoto, T., Hirayama, T., Koyama, S. (1991). Chronic motor cortex stimulation for the treatment of central pain. *Acta Neurochir Suppl (Wien)*, 52, 137-9.

Tsubokawa, T., Katayama, Y., Yamamomto, T., Hirayama, T., Koyama, S. (1993). Chronic motor cortex stimulation in patients with thalamic pain. *J Neurosurg*, 78, 393–401.

Wider, M., Ahlstrom, G. (2002). Disability after a stroke and the influence of long-term pain on everyday life. *Scand J of Caring Sciences*, 16, 302-310.

# Radiofrequency Treatments for Neuropathic Pain: Review and New Approaches

Ken-ichiro Uchida
*Department of Anesthesiology, Kurashiki Central Hospital*
*Japan*

## 1. Introduction

There are 2 types of radiofrequency treatment (RF) for neuropathic pain: thermal (continuous) RF and pulsed RF (PRF).

Thermal RF (TRF) uses a constant high-frequency electric current (100,000-500,000 Hz) to produce tissue temperatures of 45 °C or more, resulting in neuroablative thermocoagulation. Thus, TRF is a neurolytic technique that uses heat for controlled destruction of nociceptive pathways. However, the use of TRF for the management of neuropathic pain is controversial because neuroablation can lead to lasting motor deficits, neuritis, and deafferentation pain.

PRF was developed as an alternative to TRF. In PRF, the current is delivered in short pulses, and the tip temperature of the probe is adjusted so that it does not increase above 42 °C, thus avoiding lesions. PRF has been applied to treat various chronic pain conditions (Chua et al., 2011) but, the mechanisms of the analgesic action have not been studied in detail, and the optimal electrical parameters (voltage and duration) have not been established.

This chapter discusses the use of both TRF and PRF for treating neuropathic pain. We excluded treatments administered for arthropathy or discogenic pain, such as RF of the medial branch that innervates the zygapophyseal joints or that of the intervertebral disc.

The review section of this chapter critically evaluates the efficacy of TRF and PRF by discussing several randomized clinical trials (RCTs) and well-designed observational studies. Therefore, case reports also have been excluded.

We then presented our results from 2 self-controlled studies on each method.

## 2. TRF for neuropathic pain

### 2.1 Mechanism of action

The passage of low-energy, high-frequency alternating current (100,000–500,000 Hz) causes intense oscillations of tissue ions. This oscillation heats charged macromolecules, most notably proteins (Organ, 1976–1977). In TRF, heating during RF causes many cells to die rapidly if tissue temperatures reach 45 °C. Neuroablation is produced whether the electrode is placed inside the dorsal root ganglion (DRG) or onto a peripheral nerve. Above 55 °C, there is indiscriminate destruction of both small- and large-diameter myelinated fibers, accompanied by focal necrosis, hemorrhages, extensive edema, and features of Wallerian degeneration. Even with a voltage as low as 0.1 V, an electrode placed inside a DRG and heated to 67 °C results in total loss of myelinated fibers and hemorrhage (de Louw et al., 2001; Govind & Bogduk, 2010; Podhajsky et al., 2005; Smith et al., 1981).

The mode of action of RF was initially attributed to the thermocoagulation of nerve fibers, but contradictory observations (most notably that only transient sensory loss is observed in the associated dermatome, whereas the pain relief may last much longer) suggest that temperature is not the only mechanism responsible for the decrease in pain transmission (Racz & Ruiz-Lopez, 2006).

### 2.2 Treatment of neuropathic pain and its complications

#### 2.2.1 Trigeminal neuralgia

Trigeminal neuralgia is a common, idiopathic form of neuropathic pain that presents with paroxysms of pain involving 1 or more divisions of the trigeminal nerve.

TRF of the trigeminal ganglion has been used for decades to treat trigeminal neuralgia, and several large retrospective series have been conducted to evaluate the efficacy of this procedure. Taha and Tew (Taha & Tew, 1996) reevaluated the effects of TRF on trigeminal ganglion and compared the effectiveness with other surgical procedures for the treatment of trigeminal neuralgia. In this study, among the successfully completed procedures (n = 6205), complete initial pain relief was highest after TRF and microvascular decompression (MVD) (98%), whereas, glycerol rhizotomy and balloon compression relieved pain in 91% and 93% of patients, respectively. TRF had the highest success rate (98%) when considering both completion of the procedure and achievement of pain relief, whereas lowest success rates were achieved by glycerol rhizotomy (85%) and MVD (83%). The rate of pain recurrence following these percutaneous techniques was lower with TRF (20% in 9 years) than with glycerol rhizotomy (54% in 4 years) or balloon compression (21% in 2 years).

The chief disadvantages of TRF of the trigeminal ganglion was that the deliberately produces sensory loss with an unavoidable incidence of neuropathic pain in some patients (Niv & Gofeld, 2009). The most common complications and adverse effects of TRF of the trigeminal ganglion included facial numbness (98%), dysesthesia (24%), anesthesia dolorosa (1.5%), corneal anesthesia (7%), keratitis (1%), and trigeminal motor dysfunction (24%) (Rathmell, 2009). The mechanism of injury during TRF for trigeminal neuralgia may be related to injury caused during placement of the cannula or injury caused by thermal destruction during the procedure.

#### 2.2.2 DRG

TRF of DRG (TRF-DRG) is mainly used to treat persistent radicular pain. Although uncontrolled studies reported acceptable clinical efficacy, the controlled clinical data on TRF yielded variable results that depended on the pain syndrome treated and the specific mode of TRF-DRG employed (Malik & Benzon, 2008). To date, there is limited evidence for only short-term relief of cervicobrachial pain, no conclusive evidence that TRF-DRG is an effective treatment for cervicogenic headaches, and limited evidence against its use in the treatment of lumbar radicular pain.

Three prospective controlled trials have examined TRF-DRG for treating neuropathic pain stemming from cervical DRG.

Van Kleef et al. (van Kleef et al., 1996) divided the patients with intractable chronic cervicobrachial pain into 2 treatment groups: 9 patients underwent TRF of the cervical DRG at 67 °C, whereas 11 underwent sham treatment. Patients were evaluated before the procedure and 8 weeks after it. Eight patients in the thermal RF group (88.8%) and 2 patients (18.1%) in the sham group reported pain relief. Regarding side effects of TRF, 7 patients treated with TRF noticed a faint burning sensation in the treated dermatome that subsided within 3 weeks after treatment.

Slappendel et al. (Slappendel et al., 1997) conducted second RCT involving TRF of the cervical DRG in patients with cervicobrachial pain. They compared 32 patients who received TRF-DRG at 67 °C with 29 patients who received TRF-DRG at 40 °C, which could not produce neuroablative thermocoagulation. No statistically significant difference in pain scores was found between the 2 groups. Neuritis was reported in the TRF-DRG at 67 °C group (18.8%) and TRF-DRG at 40 °C group (17.2%) 6 weeks after TRF-DRG. Moreover, a few patients reported motor disturbances with a decreased pinch force 3 months after treatment.

A trial by Haspeslagh et al. (Haspeslagh et al., 2006) included 30 patients with cervicogenic headache. Patients were randomized to 2 groups. One group (n = 15) was treated by TRF of cervical facet joints, followed by TRF of the cervical DRG at 67 °C if necessary, whereas the second group (n = 15) was treated by injections of a steroid and a local anesthetic into the greater occipital nerve, followed by transcutaneous electrical nerve stimulation (TENS) if necessary. There was no significant difference in the success rate between the 2 treatments, and the authors concluded that sequential TRF of facet joints and DRG had similar efficacy to local steroid and anesthetic injection, followed by TENS.

There have been no prospective controlled trials on TRF of the thoracic DRG.

Stolker et al. (Stolker et al., 1994) conducted a prospective uncontrolled trial using TRF of the thoracic DRG at 67 °C to treat 45 patients afflicted with thoracic segmental pain. They reported that 91% patients obtained > 50% pain relief at 2 months and that 78% continued to experience pain relief for 13 to 46 months. A smaller number of patients (13.3%) reported a transient burning pain in the corresponding dermatome that subsided within 3 weeks.

There is only 1 prospective controlled trial on the clinical efficacy of TRF of the lumbar DRG. A trial by Geurts et al. (Geurts et al., 2003) included 83 patients with chronic lumbosacral pain; 45 patients underwent TRF-DRG at 67 °C, whereas 38 underwent sham treatment. After 3 months, 16% patients treated with TRF-DRG and 25% of sham-treated patients reported a decrease in lumbosacral pain ($P = 0.43$). Adverse events and complications, such as treatment-related pain, changes in sensation, or loss of motor function, did not differ between the treatment groups. They concluded that TRF was not an effective treatment for chronic lumbosacral radicular pain and stressed that such patients would attain little benefit from TRF-DRG.

Whereas the clinical efficacy of TRF was confirmed for some types of neuropathic pain, each of these studies has limitations, particularly small sample numbers and short-term follow-up. In their review, Malik and Benzon (Malik & Benzon, 2008) concluded that larger-scale, longer-term, controlled clinical trials are required to clearly establish the efficacy of TRF-DRG for different types of neuropathic pain, particularly pain originating from thoracic DRG.

#### 2.2.3 Sympathetic ganglia

Although systematic reviews have found no tangible evidence supporting the benefit of sympathectomy for the management of neuropathic pain, TRF of the stellate, thoracic, and lumbar sympathetic ganglia has been used for treatment of neuropathic pain arising from sympathetic ganglia dysfunction such as complex regional pain syndrome. However, evidence for the therapeutic efficacy of TRF, is limited to small case series. RCTs are needed to validate the efficacy of TRF for these syndromes and to define measurable and reproducible end points for it.

## 3. Neuropathic pain treatment by combined TRF and glucocorticoids

### 3.1 Background

TRF is controversial because of its neurodestructive nature (Bogduk, 2006; de Louw et al., 2001; Podhajsky et al., 2005; Smith et al., 1981; Uematsu et al., 1974). Heat lesions produced by TRF causing neural destruction have sequelae similar to other forms of neural injury. Even with proper technique, TRF is associated with sensory loss and the onset of neuropathic pain. Although the frequency of these complications is minimized by the proper use of sensory and motor stimulation trials to isolate somatosensory and motor axons before lesion, injury to adjacent nerves can easily occur (Rathmell, 2009). Glucocorticoids have been used to treat neuropathic pain for many years, and they do effectively alleviate acute and continued postoperative pain by suppressing inflammatory mediators and glial activation, resulting in decreased nociceptive activity, sympathetic sprouting, and central neuropathic changes such as central sensitization (Romundstad & Stubhaug, 2007). We suggest that the effect of glucocorticoids could be additive to that of TRF and that glucocorticoids might avert pain associated with neuroinflammation after RF lesioning.

### 3.2 Methods

#### 3.2.1 Patients

Fourteen patients (7 females, 7 males) with refractory neuropathic pain from postherpetic neuralgia were included in this study. Median age was 70.5 years (interquartile range, 69.3–71.8 years). The median pain duration was 9.0 months (interquartile range, 7.0–13.5 months).

Patients were selected to undergo TRF of the thoracic paravertebral nerve (TRF-TPN) combined with glucocorticoid according to the following criteria: (1) the presence of radiating pain in the thoracic region following herpes zoster; (2) no response to conventional treatments such as anti-inflammatory drugs, antidepressants, anticonvulsants, opioid analgesics, and topical capsaicin; (3) at least 6 months of conventional treatment; (4) temporary positive response (100% pain relief) to TPN block using local anesthetics and glucocorticoids (conventional NB) at each painful dermatome; and (5) pain severe enough to disturb sleep.

Exclusion criteria were as follows: (1) MRI showing acute pathology; (2) history of adverse reactions to local anesthetics or glucocorticoids; or (3) coagulation disorders, or use of anticoagulants.

After we provided complete information on the RF technique and its possible benefits, risks, and side effects, the patients gave verbal informed consent for the procedure.

### 3.2.2 Conventional paravertebral nerve block

In the first part of this study, conventional nerve block (NB) was achieved using a local anesthetic and glucocorticoid, and the duration of pain relief was recorded.

The duration of pain relief was defined as the number of days after the treatment until the pain intensity returned to the level experienced before treatment.

The level at which conventional NB was administered was determined by the affected dermatome, the degree of tenderness under the rib using fluoroscopy with a C-arm, and the effect of the intercostal NB.

Conventional NB was performed using a 22-gauge, 80-mm needle under real-time fluoroscopy with a C-arm by the laterodorsal approach (Uchida, 2009). We administered 1.5 ml of 2% mepivacaine as the local anesthetic and 2 mg of betamethasone (Rinderon®, Shionogi, Osaka, Japan) as the glucocorticoid.

### 3.2.3 Radiofrequency procedures

Four to eight weeks after assessment of the effect of conventional NB, TRF-TPN was administered in the same manner as the previous conventional NB. In the TRF procedure, the electrode (22-gauge 99-mm needle with 4-mm bare tip, TFW 22G × 99 mm®, Hakko, Japan) was used instead of a 22-gauge, 80-mm needle. Once the electrode was positioned, the electrode stylet was replaced with a thermocouple electrode. We tested whether the thermocouple electrode was placed in the physiologically correct location by applying 100-Hz stimulation of the needle tip. We initially set the voltage at 0 V, and then gradually increased it until the patient felt a tingling sensation. If a tingling sensation in the corresponding dermatome was reported at a voltage of < 0.5 V, the electrode was assumed to be in the correct position. After verifying that the needle was in the correct position, 1.5 ml of 2% mepivacaine and 2 mg of betamethasone were administered.

Five minutes later, TRF-TPN was applied at 90 °C and duration of 90 seconds under control of a generator (Neuro Therm JK 3™ system, Croydon, Surrey, UK) with an automatic temperature control mode to avoid excessive elevation of temperature. After therapy, the number of days of pain relief and the complications resulting from TRF-TPN were recorded.

## 3.3 Results

### 3.3.1 Primary outcomes

The duration of pain relief after TRF was significantly longer than that after conventional NB ($P < 0.0001$, Kaplan–Meier analysis and the log-rank statistic) (Figure 1).

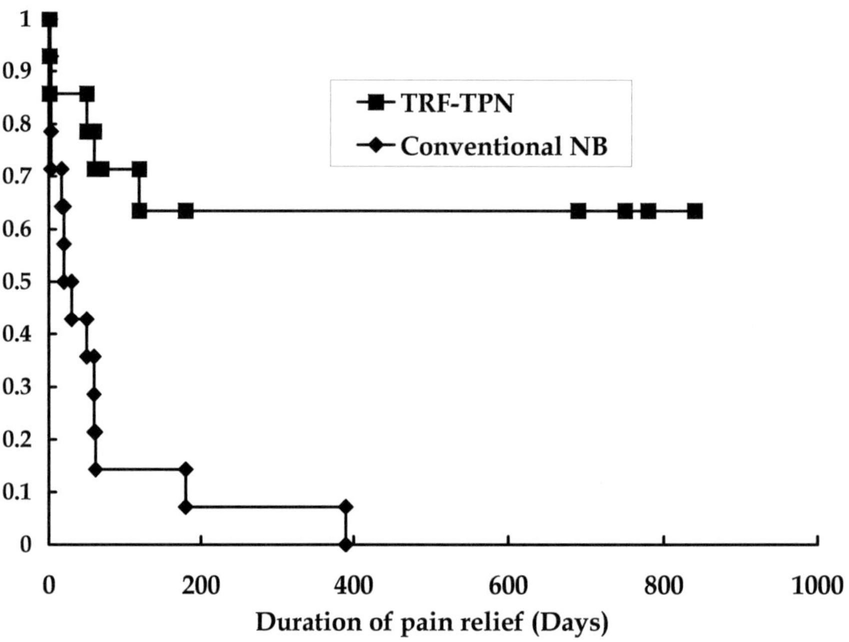


Fig. 1. Analgesic effect of conventional NB vs. TRF of TPN.

Kaplan-Meier graphs depicting the cumulative proportions of patients who reported pain relief following conventional NB or TRF-TPN. Censored values represent patients whose pain returned to pretreatment levels. The vertical axis indicates cumulative proportion of patients reporting pain relief.

### 3.3.2 Secondary outcome

The mean electrical sensory stimulation threshold before TRF-TPN was 0.20 ± 0.14 V (mean ± SD) at 100 Hz and 0.20 V at 3 Hz (median, interquartile range: 0.10–0.35 V). The impedance after therapy (local anesthetic and glucocorticoid injection + TRF) was significantly lower than that measured before TRF (before TRF: 637.9 ± 182.4 Ω; after therapy: 511.6 ± 79.3 Ω; mean ± SD, $P = 0.0045$ by paired t-test).

In all cases, hypoesthesia increased in the corresponding dermatome after TRF. No major complications, such as anesthesia dolorosa and burning pain, were reported after the procedure, and no patient claimed that their pain had increased after the procedure.

## 3.4 Discussion

Controversy has arisen over the use of TRF for the management of nonmalignant neuropathic pain because of its potential for neurodestruction, which could lead to motor deficits, neuritis, and deafferentation pain. Van Kleef et al. (Van Kleef et al., 1995) suggested that the potential hazard of nonspecific neural destruction after treatment with TRF-DRG might actually intensify symptoms by inducing deafferentation pain. Therefore, they insisted that TRF-DRG was not suitable for neuropathic pain syndromes with sensory loss due to nerve damage, such as postthoracotomy pain, postherpetic neuralgia, and postmastectomy syndrome, and that TRF-DRG should be restricted to purely nociceptive pain syndromes.

Peripheral nerve destruction caused by TRF has paradoxical effects on neuropathic pain. It is believed that the therapeutic effect of TRF is achieved by a partial nerve lesion to nociceptive afferents (Bogduk, 2006). On the other hand, minor nerve injury can sometimes produce devastating pain, whereas modest or diffuse deafferentation does not (Devor et al. 2006). The cause of this effect has not been elucidated. In a clinical study, it was suggested that even long-standing central sensitization can be reversed quickly when the peripheral input is removed (Gracely et al., 1992). Therefore we believe that TRF is an acceptable treatment modality for neuropathic pain.

We used TRF-TPN for postherpetic neuralgia instead of TRF-DRG in this case series. TRF-TPN has an simpler surgical approach than TRF-DRG and thus a lower probability of injuring the radicular artery, an event that may induce serious neurologic complications, including brain and spinal cord infarction and death (Uchida, 2009) .

We reported previously that repeated administration of TRF-TPN combined with glucocorticoid administration decreased pain and improved the quality of life in patients with the refractory neuropathic pain of postmastectomy syndrome (Uchida, 2009).

Although the use of glucocorticoids for NB is also controversial, glucocorticoids are usually coadministered with a local anesthetic. Pro-inflammatory cytokines secreted at or near the site of nerve injury are involved in the development and maintenance of central sensitization and neuropathic pain (Romundstad & Stubhaug, 2007).

The lesions produced by the RF energy are well-demarcated areas of coagulative necrosis surrounded by inflammatory cell infiltrate and hemorrhage. This inflammatory response can lead to increased tenderness, pain, and limited movement after TRF (Dobrogowski et al., 2005). Glucocorticoids are known to suppress pro-inflammatory cytokines (such as TNFα and IL-1β) and induce the expression of anti-inflammatory cytokines (such as IL-10). Moreover, there is convincing evidence for acute analgesic and antihyperalgesic effects of glucocorticoids after surgery in humans and experimental injuries in animal models (Romundstad & Stubhaug, 2007).

The duration of pain relief was significantly longer after TRF-TPN treatment than after conventional NB in this self-controlled study, and few serious side effects were reported despite the increased hypoesthesia. Van Kleef et al. (van Kleef et al., 1995) evaluated the effectiveness of TRF-DRG (67 °C, 60 s) on patients presenting with chronic thoracic pain and reported significantly better short-term and long-term pain relief. However, in their report, 14 (33%) out of 43 patients experienced a mild burning pain in the treated dermatome for some days following treatment. In our previous report, 3 patients experienced no transient burning pain after 21 successive TRF-TPN despite the high temperature and repetition (Uchida, 2009). Dobrogowski et al. (Dobrogowski et al., 2005) found that TRF with methylprednisolone administration to the lumbar medial branch tended to decrease the frequency of postoperative pain.

Although the site and extent of treatment were different as well as the degree of the effect of glucocorticoid remains unclear, these results suggests that glucocorticoids can decrease the pain related to neural injury after TRF.

## 4. Pulsed radiofrequency treatment for neuropathic pain

### 4.1 Mechanism of action

Two theories have been proposed to explain the analgesic effects of PRF.

One is that pain relief depends on the rapidly changing electric fields (Sluijter, 1998); the other is that PRF produces brief heat bursts at temperatures in the range associated with destructive heat lesions (Cosman & Cosman, 2005). It is not known, however, if these transient heat bursts do have an ablative effect (Chua et al., 2011).

Secondary effects on the nervous system after PRF application have been studied in animal models (Erdine et al., 2009; Erdine et al., 2005; Hamann et al., 2006; Higuchi et al., 2002; Podhajsky et al., 2005; Protasoni et al., 2009; Tun et al., 2009; Van Zundert et al., 2005). These studies reported increased c-Fos expression in the dorsal horn (Higuchi et al., 2002; Van Zundert et al., 2005), increased expression of activating transcription factor 3 (Hamann et al., 2006), and morphological changes in the DRG or the peripheral nerve (Erdine et al., 2009; Erdine et al., 2005; Podhajsky et al., 2005; Protasoni et al., 2009; Tun et al., 2009).

### 4.2 Treatment of neuropathic pain and treatment complications

#### 4.2.1 Trigeminal neuralgia

For trigeminal neuralgia, the therapeutic efficacy of PRF has neither surpassed nor equaled TRF. Erdine et al. (Erdine et al., 2007) compared the efficacy of TRF with PRF of the trigeminal ganglion in patients with idiopathic trigeminal neuralgia. Significant pain reductions were reported in all patients treated with TRF (n = 20), whereas only 2 of 20 patients in the PRF treatment group reported pain reduction. Five of the 20 TRF patients and 3 of 20 PRF patients reported moderate headache for 24 h. There was mild hypoesthesia and paresthesia in all patients from the TRF group. Anesthesia dolorosa occurred in 1 patient from the TRF group and medical treatment was given. They concluded that PRF, unlike TRF, was not an effective treatment method for idiopathic trigeminal neuralgia.

#### 4.2.2 DRG

Two RCTs have examined PRF of DRG for neuropathic pain (Simopoulos *et al.*, 2008; Van Zundert *et al.*, 2007). These studies presented limited evidence that PRF of the cervical DRG could produce short-term relief of cervical radicular pain; however, there is limited evidence against its use existed in treatment of lumbar radicular pain (Malik & Benzon, 2008).

Van Zundert et al. (Van Zundert et al., 2007) compared PRF of the cervical DRG to sham treatment at 3 months after treatment; PRF of the cervical DRG showed significantly better outcome on both the global perceived effect (> 50% improvement) index and visual analog scale (20-point pain reduction).

Simopoulos et al. (Simopoulos et al., 2008) randomly divided patients with lumbosacral radicular pain into 2 groups; 1 group was treated with PRF only, whereas the second group was treated first with PRF and then with TRF at the maximum tolerated temperature. There was no significant difference in the response rate or in the average decline in VAS between the 2 groups. Survival curves showed that for both treatment groups experienced a steep loss in the analgesic effect between 2 and 4 months after the procedure. By the 8$^{th}$ month, the vast majority of patients relapsed to baseline pain intensity.

Malik and Benzon (Malik & Benzon, 2008) reviewed published articles on PRF-DRG and concluded that none of the studies reported any significant side effects or complications.

However, Sluijter (Sluijter, 2001) divided the postoperative observational period after PRF procedure into four phases and found that the second phase was associated with the highest post-procedure discomfort, which lasted up to 3 weeks.

## 5. Low-voltage PRF treatment for radicular neuropathic pain

### 5.1 Background

The clinical effects of PRF have been examined for various regions and pain conditions using voltage outputs of 20–45 V. There are no standardized criteria for the voltage output of PRF, except that voltage should not be sufficient to increase temperature above 42 °C. However, rapid temperature spikes above 42 °C were observed during PRF bursts of 45 V, occasionally reaching the lethal temperature range of 45–50 °C or more (Cosman & Cosman, 2005). These rapid temperature spikes might induce microscopic tissue damage, leading to a period of discomfort after PRF, and induce antinociceptive action.

To avoid rapid temperature spikes, we used low-voltage PRF (L-PRF) where the voltage output is only 5 V. This section will describe the first reported effects of L-PRF for radicular neuropathic pain using a self-controlled design.

### 5.2 Materials and methods

#### 5.2.1 Patients

This study was approved by the institutional review board of the institution where our study was performed, and patients provided written informed consent for participation. The basic demographic and clinical characteristics of the patients are listed in Table 1. Patients were subgrouped according to treatment sites as cervical (C), thoracic (T), and lumbar (L).

| | Age (years)* | Female/Male | Duration of Pain (months)* | Etiology |
|---|---|---|---|---|
| C | 49 (49-55) | 10/2 | 14 (10-21) | Cervicobrachialgia |
| T | 70 (68-72) | 3/7 | 6 (5-6) | Postherpetic neuralgia |
| L | 70 (65-79) | 5/3 | 74 (14-80) | Degenerative spondylosis |

*Median (Interquartile range)

Table 1. Characteristics of the Subjects

Patients were selected for this study according to the following criteria: (1) chronic unilateral radicular pain of at least 3 months' duration that could not be adequately controlled with oral medications; (2) average pain intensity higher than 30 mm as measured on a 100 mm VAS; (3) temporary positive response (100% reduction of pain) more than twice to C, T, or L DRG block with local anesthetics and glucocorticoids under fluoroscopy; and (4) return of pain intensity to baseline after temporary relief resulting from C, T, or L DRG block.

Exclusion criteria were as follows: (1) MRI showing acute pathology; (2) history of adverse reactions to local anesthetics or glucocorticoids; or (3) history of cancer, myelopathy, diabetes mellitus, psychotherapeutic management, coagulation disorders, or use of anticoagulants.

### 5.2.2 Conventional NB procedures

Conventional NB and L-PRF of C, T, and L- DRG were performed using a 22-gauge needle under real-time fluoroscopy with a C-arm as described by Gauci (Gauci, 2004).

After fluoroscopy confirmed that the needle tip was positioned correctly, 0.2 ml of iohexol (Omnipaque 240®; Daiichi-Sankyo, Tokyo, Japan) was injected to guard against venous uptake and false-negative responses. If the contrast dye was washed out by blood flow, the needle was removed and reintroduced. Thereafter, 0.5 ml of 2% mepivacaine as the local anesthetic and 0.5 ml of 0.4% betamethasone (Rinderon®; Shionogi, Osaka, Japan) were administered.

Four to eight weeks after assessment of the effect of conventional NB, patients were treated by L-PRF.

### 5.2.3 L-PRF procedure

L-PRF was performed under fluoroscopy with a C-arm in the same manner as conventional NB. For L-PRF, an RF needle (22-gauge 99-mm needle with 4-mm bare tip, TFW 22G × 99 mm®, Hakko, Japan) was used instead of the 22-gauge injection needle used for conventional NB. After optimizing the position of the needle, we tested whether the thermocouple electrode was placed in the physiologically correct location by applying 100-Hz stimulation to the needle tip using a generator (Neuro Therm JK 3™ system; Neuro Therm, Croydon, Surrey, United Kingdom). If a tingling sensation was obtained at a voltage of < 0.5 V at 100-Hz stimulation, the electrode was assumed to be in the correct position. Each threshold was measured twice and the average was obtained. After the 100-Hz stimulation threshold was determined, we measured the stimulation threshold at 3 Hz that was required to induce throbbing and touch-like sensations in a similar manner and impedance.

Ten seconds after the measurement, L-PRF was initiated. The L-PRF protocol consisted of 20-ms radiofrequency current bursts at 2 Hz for 180 s with a generator (Neuro Therm JK 3™ system). The oscillation frequency of the alternating current was 500 kHz, which is generated by a voltage of 5 V. During 1 cycle, the active phase of 20 ms was followed by a silent period of 480 ms to allow dissipation of the generated heat.

Throughout the L-PRF, the current output, voltage, and tip temperature were recorded every 30 s.

Ten seconds after L-PRF, the electrical stimulation thresholds at 100 Hz and 3 Hz, as well as the impedance were reevaluated. Following completion of L-PRF, 0.5 ml of 2% mepivacaine and 0.5 ml of 0.4% betamethasone were administered through the RF needle into the nerve. The dosages of the local anesthetic and glucocorticoid were the same for both the conventional NB and L-PRF groups.

After conventional NB and L-PRF, the number of days of pain relief was recorded. The duration of pain relief was defined as the number of days after therapy until the pain intensity returned to the baseline level experienced before the therapy.

### 5.3 Results

#### 5.3.1 Primary outcomes

The duration of pain relief after L-PRF was significantly longer than that after conventional NB for treating all target sites (C, T, and L DRG) ($P < 0.05$, Kaplan-Meier analysis and the log rank statistic) (Figure 2, 3, and 4).

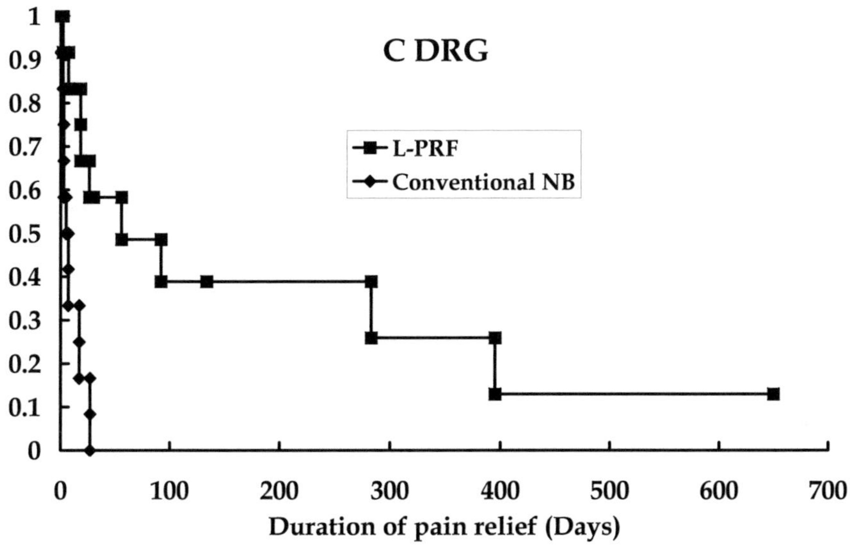


Fig. 2. Analgesic effect of conventional NB vs. L-PRF of C DRG

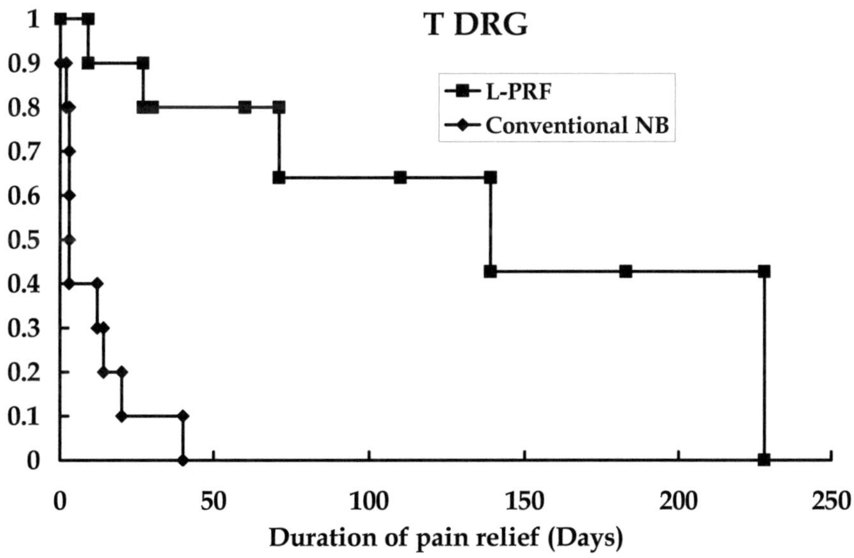


Fig. 3. Analgesic effect of conventional NB vs. L-PRF of T DRG

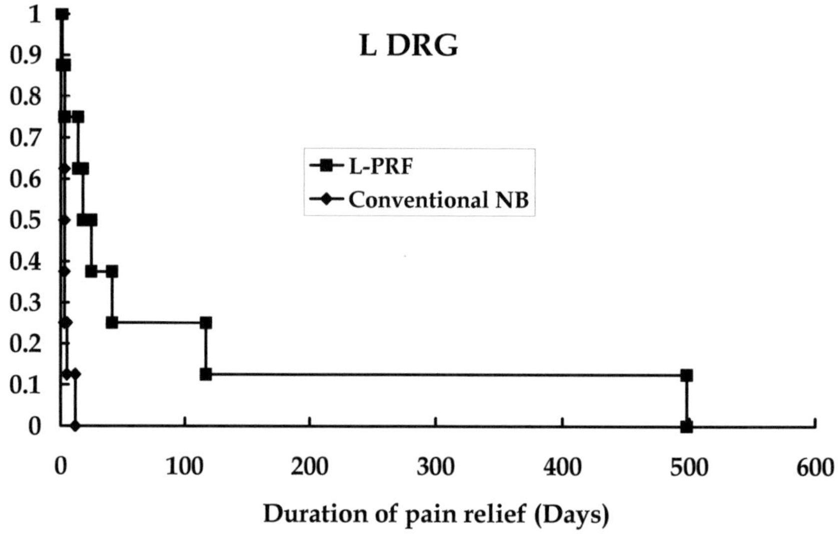


Fig. 4. Analgesic effect of conventional NB vs. L-PRF of L DRG

Kaplan-Meier graphs depicting the cumulative proportions of patients who experienced pain relief for a given period after conventional NB or L-PRF of C (Fig. 2), T (Fig. 3), and L (Fig. 4) DRG revealed that patients treated by L-PRF exhibited a much longer analgesic response. Censored values in these plots represent patients who experienced the same level of pain as before therapy. Vertical axes indicate the cumulative proportions of patients experiencing pain relief at that time.

### 5.3.2 Secondary outcome

The secondary outcomes measured included voltage, current, and temperature profiles during L-PRF (Table 2) as well as the measurements of electrical sensory stimulation thresholds at 100 Hz and 3 Hz and impedance values before and after L-PRF (Table 3) for patients treated by L-PRF of C, T, or L DRG.

| | 0 | 30 | 60 | 90 | 120 | 150 | 180 |
|---|---|---|---|---|---|---|---|
| C | | | | | | | |
| Voltage [V] | 5.0 (0.0) | 5.0 (0.0) | 5.0 (0.0) | 5.0 (0.0) | 5.0 (0.0) | 5.0 (0.0) | 5.0 (0.0) |
| Current [mA] | 20.0 (5.0) | 17.5(5.0) | 17.5 (5.0) | 17.5 (5.0) | 17.5 (5.0) | 17.5 (5.0) | 17.5 (5.0) |
| Temperature [°C] | 38.0 (0.8) | 40.0 (1.8) | 40.0 (1.8) | 40.0 (1.8) | 40.0 (1.5) | 40.0 (1.3) | 40.5 (2.3) |
| T | | | | | | | |
| Voltage [V] | 5.0 (0.8) | 5.0 (0.0) | 5.0 (0.0) | 5.0 (0.0) | 5.0 (0.0) | 5.0 (0.0) | 5.0 (0.0) |
| Current [mA] | 15.0 (3.8) | 15.0 (3.8) | 15.0 (3.8) | 15.0 (3.8) | 15.0 (3.8) | 15.0 (3.8) | 15.0 (3.8) |
| Temperature [°C] | 38.5 (1.0) | 40.0 (1.0) | 41.0 (1.8) | 41.0 (1.8) | 41.0 (1.0) | 41.0 (1.0) | 41.5 (1.0) |
| L | | | | | | | |
| Voltage [V] | 5.0 (0.0) | 5.0 (0.0) | 5.0 (0.0) | 5.0 (0.0) | 5.0 (0.0) | 5.0 (0.0) | 5.0 (0.0) |
| Current [mA] | 20.0 (5.0) | 20.0 (2.5) | 20.0 (5.0) | 20.0 (2.5) | 20.0 (2.5) | 20.0 (2.5) | 20.0 (5.0) |
| Temperature [°C] | 38.0 (1.5) | 41.0 (2.0) | 42.0 (0.5) | 42.0 (1.0) | 42.0 (0.0) | 42.0 (0.0) | 42.0 (0.0) |

The median and interquartile ranges are presented in each cell of this table.

Table 2. Electrical and temperature profiles during 180-s L-PRF

The electrical sensory stimulation threshold at 100 Hz and 3 Hz after L-PRF was significantly higher than that before treatment (C and L DRG group: $P < 0.05$ by paired t-test, T DRG group: $P < 0.05$ by Wilcoxon's signed rank test). The impedance after L-PRF was significantly lower than that before treatment in all groups ($P < 0.05$, paired t-test, respectively) (Table 3).

| | 100 Hz [V] | | 3 Hz [V] | | Impedance [Ω] | |
|---|---|---|---|---|---|---|
| | Baseline | After | Baseline | After | Baseline | After |
| C | 0.26 ± 0.14 | 0.51 ± 0.21* | 0.50 ± 0.47 | 0.62 ± 0.39* | 505.8 ± 77.6 | 448.0 ± 63.6* |
| T | 0.19 (0.13–0.35) | 0.35 (0.12–0.49)* | 0.21 (0.20–0.33) | 0.34 (0.31–0.54)* | 582.2 ± 88.2 | 492.0 ± 100.3* |
| L | 0.15 ± 0.11 | 0.35 ± 0.18* | 0.24 ± 0.19 | 0.35 ± 0.16* | 586.1 ± 144.7 | 441.3 ± 74.5* |

Values are expressed as mean ± SD or median (interquartile range). *$P < 0.05$, versus baseline values.

Table 3. Electrical sensory stimulation thresholds at 100 Hz and 3 Hz and impedance before and after L-PRF

### 5.4 Discussion

In this study, PRF was administered at low voltage (5 V) to avoid temperature spikes that might induce heat lesions and lead to a period of discomfort after treatment. The calculated and measured heat spikes during PRF should be proportional to $V(peak)^2/2R$ (resistance), where V (peak) is the peak RF voltage on the electrode (Cosman & Cosman, 2005). Therefore heat spikes in this study were about 1/16-81 in comparison with that at 20-45 V. Although the actual tissue temperature around the electrode could not be measured, it was assumed that the heat spikes by L-PRF treatment were suppressed enough.

In this study, the duration of pain relief after L-PRF treatment was significantly longer than that after conventional NB. Although it is difficult to compare our results with those following conventional PRF-DRG because the study protocols are different, this improved efficacy of L-PRF seems correlates with the results following conventional PRF-DRG (Chua et al., 2011).

Moreover, we applied 100-Hz and 3-Hz electrical stimulation before and immediately after L-PRF and recorded the changes in electrical sensory stimulation thresholds to detect the immediate effect of L-PRF on nerve excitability. Despite the significant decrease in the impedance after L-PRF, the electrical sensory stimulation thresholds at 100 Hz and 3 Hz were significantly higher immediately after L-PRF. We cannot explain the relationship between the elevation in sensory stimulation threshold and the prolonged pain relief after L-PRF. This observed decline in sensory perception may reflect the prompt analgesic effect of L-PRF, which raises the possibility that this phenomenon induces long-term changes in gene expression that underlie neuronal plasticity (Van Zundert et al., 2005).

There is no evidence to suggest that L-PRF and conventional PRF work through different mechanisms. Two parameters related to rapidly changing electric fields are keys to the change in neuronal transmission: temperature and electrical pattern.

The median tip temperature of the electrode ranged from 38 °C to 42 °C in our study. Heating a nerve to a relatively low temperature (40-45 °C) has been reported to block conduction along the nerve, but only temporarily (Brodkey et al., 1964). These reports lend support to the possibility that L-PRF has a transient inhibitory effect on sensory transmission.

The electrical pattern of L-PRF consisted of 2 distinct phases: bursts of 2 Hz and oscillating current of 500 kHz.

Bursts of 2 Hz are at almost the same frequency as that used for TENS. Munglani (Munglani, 1999) suggested that PRF works in a manner similar to TENS, activating both spinal and supraspinal mechanisms that may decrease sensory perception. Nerve stimulation at 1-2 Hz was shown to induce long-term depression (LTD) of synaptic transmission in the spinal cord (Pockett, 1995, Sandkühler et al., 1997). De Col and Maihöfner (De Col & Maihöfner, 2008) reported that sensory decline was induced after transcutaneous electrical stimulation at 0.5 Hz or 20 Hz and that the underlying mechanisms might involve higher sensory integration centers such as the thalamus, primary somatosensory cortex (S1), secondary somatosensory cortex (S2), and surrounding somatosensory association cortices that process noxious and innocuous stimuli.

Cosman and Cosman (Cosman & Cosman, 2005) calculated that the rapid oscillation in transmembrane potential in response to a 500-kHz current would induce transmembrane rectification of neuronal currents, which might also cause LTD as well as depolarizing pulses at 1-2 Hz. In this case, both temporal phases of current oscillation might induce LTD and thereby decrease afferent pain transmission.

This pulsed stimulus pattern might also induce secondary effects in the nervous system, such as enhancement of the descending noradrenergic and serotonergic inhibitory pathways (Hagiwara et al., 2009), that modulate neuropathic pain. Furthermore, histological analyses revealed changes in neuronal morphology following PRF (Erdine et al., 2009; Erdine et al., 2005; Podhajsky et al., 2005; Protasoni et al., 2009; Tun et al., 2009), which may alter the electronic properties of sensory neurons and potentially interrupt normal afferent signaling to the spinal cords.

Although the applied site and the electric profiles of PRF were different, it is possible that our observation was related to these mechanisms.

To date, PRF has not achieved the clinical efficacy of TRF (Govind & Bogduk, 2010). However, PRF has a principal advantage over TRF. By minimizing structural damage to nontarget axons through heat dissipation, PRF is associated with fewer side effects. From this perspective, L-PRF might be an attractive alternative treatment, if L-PRF surpasses the clinical efficacy of conventional NB and does indeed induce fewer or less severe thermal lesions than conventional PRF or TRF.

In conclusion, L-PRF of the DRG resulted in significantly longer pain relief compared with conventional NB in patients with chronic radicular pain. To elucidate the mode of action of PRF, further research is needed. Furthermore, the optimal stimulus parameters must be determined to improve analgesic efficacy and safety.

## 6. Conclusion

This chapter presented evidence demonstrating the clinical efficacy of RF for the treatment of neuropathic pain. We also presented 2 preliminary studies showing that TRF combined with glucocorticoids and L-PRF are useful, and possibly safer, treatments for neuropathic pain. These studies are preliminary and a lot of work needs to be done before the mechanism of action and most effective electric parameters are defined.

Although chronic neuropathic pain is a clinical challenge, radiofrequency treatments have several benefits including relative safety and technical simplicity. If pharmacological treatment and conventional NB have failed, RF might be a valuable alternative for patients with refractory neuropathic pain.

## 7. Acknowledgement

The author acknowledges Mayumi Ikeda and Kyoko Miyake of the Anesthesiology Department at Kurashiki Central Hospital for assistance in data collection.

## 8. References

Bogduk, N. (2006). Pulsed radiofrequency. *Pain Med,* Vol.7, No.5, (2006 Sep/Oct), pp. (396-407), ISSN 1526-2375.

Brodkey, JS., Miyazaki, Y., Ervin, FR. & Mark, VH. (1964). Reversible heat lesions with radiofrequency current. A method of stereotactic localization. *J Neurosurg,* Vol.21, (1964 Jan), pp.(49-53), ISSN 0022-3085.

Chua, NH., Vissers, KC. & Sluijter, ME. (2011). Pulsed radiofrequency treatment in interventional pain management: mechanisms and potential indications-a review. *Acta Neurochir,* Vol.153, No.4, (2011 Apr), pp.(763-771), ISSN 0001-6268.

Cosman, ER., Jr. & Cosman, ER., Sr. (2005). Electric and thermal field effects in tissue around radiofrequency electrodes. *Pain Med,* Vol.6, No.6, (2005 Nov-Dec), pp.(405-24), ISSN 1526-2375.

Devor, M. (2006). Peripheral nerve generators of neuropathic pain. In: *Emerging strategies for the treatment of neuropathic pain,* Campbell, JN., Basbaum, AI., Dray, A., Dubner, R., Dworkin, RH., & Sang, CN., pp.(37-68), IASP Press, ISBN 0-931092-61-2, Seattle, USA.

De Col, R. & Maihöfner, C. (2008). Centrally mediated sensory decline induced by differential c-fiber stimulation. *Pain,* Vol. 138, No. 3, (2008 Sep), pp.(556-64), ISSN 0304-3959.

De Louw, AJ., Vles, HS., Freling, G., Herpers, MJ., Arends, JW. & Kleef, M. (2001). The morphological effects of a radio frequency lesion adjacent to the dorsal root ganglion (RF-DRG)-an experimental study in the goat. *Eur J Pain,* Vol.5, No.2, pp. (169-74), ISSN 1090-3801.

Dobrogowski, J., Wrzosek, A. & Wordliczek, J. (2005). Radiofrequency denervation with or without addition of pentoxifylline or methylprednisolone for chronic lumbar zygapophysial joint pain. *Pharmacol Rep,* Vol.57, No.4, pp.(475-80), ISSN 1734-1140.

Erdine, S., Bilir, A., Cosman, ER. & Cosman, ER., Jr. (2009). Ultrastructural changes in axons following exposure to pulsed radiofrequency fields. *Pain Pract,* Vol.9, No.6, (2009 Nov-Dec), pp.(407-17), ISSN 1530-7085.

Erdine, S., Ozyalcin, NS., Cimen, A., Celik, M., Talu, GK. & Disci, R. (2007). Comparison of pulsed radiofrequency with conventional radiofrequency in the treatment of idiopathic trigeminal neuralgia. *Eur J Pain,* Vol.11, No.3, (2007 Apr), pp.(309-313), ISSN 1090-3801.

Erdine, S., Yucel, A., Cimen, A., Aydin, S., Sav, A. & Bilir, A. (2005). Effects of pulsed versus conventional radiofrequency current on rabbit dorsal root ganglion morphology. *Eur J Pain,* Vol.9, No.3, (2005 Jun), pp.(251-6), ISSN 1090-3801.

Gauci, C.A. (2004). *Manual of RF Techniques,* FlivoPress SA, ISBN 3-909 441-03-3, Meggen, Switzerland.

Geurts, JW., Van Wijk, RM., Wynne, H J., Hammink, E., Buskens, E., Lousberg, R., Knape, JT. & Groen, GJ. (2003). Radiofrequency lesioning of dorsal root ganglia for chronic lumbosacral radicular pain: A randomised, double-blind, controlled trial. *Lancet,* Vol.361, No.9351, (2003 Jan), pp.(21-6), ISSN 0140-6736.

Govind, J., Bogduk, N. (2010). Neurolytic Blockade for Noncancer Pain, In: *Bonica's Management of Pain, 4th edition.* Fishman, SM., Ballantyne, JC., & Rathmell, JP. (Eds.), pp.(1467-1485), Lippincott Williams & Wilkins, ISBN 978-0-7817-6827-6, Philadelphia, USA.

Gracely, RH., Lynch, SA. & Bennett, GJ. (1992). Painful neuropathy: Altered central processing maintained dynamically by peripheral input. *Pain,* Vol.51, No.2, (1992 Nov), pp.(175-94), ISSN 0304-3959.

Hagiwara, S., Iwasaka, H., Takeshima, N. & Noguchi, T. (2009). Mechanisms of analgesic action of pulsed radiofrequency on adjuvant-induced pain in the rat: Roles of descending adrenergic and serotonergic systems. *Eur J Pain,* Vol.13, No.3, (2009 Mar), pp. (249-52), ISSN 1090-3801.

Hamann, W., Abou-Sherif, S., Thompson, S. & Hall, S. (2006). Pulsed radiofrequency applied to dorsal root ganglia causes a selective increase in ATF3 in small neurons. *Eur J Pain,* Vol.10, No.2, (2006 Feb), pp.( 171-6), ISSN 1090-3801.

Haspeslagh, SR., Van Suijlekom, HA., Lame, IE., Kessels, AG., Van Kleef, M. & Weber, WE. (2006). Randomised controlled trial of cervical radiofrequency lesions as a treatment for cervicogenic headache [ISRCTN07444684]. *BMC Anesthesiol,* Vol.6, No.1, (2006 Feb), pp.(1-11), ISSN 1471-2253.

Higuchi, Y., Nashold, BS., Jr., Sluijter, M., Cosman, E. & Pearlstein, RD. (2002). Exposure of the dorsal root ganglion in rats to pulsed radiofrequency currents activates dorsal horn lamina I and II neurons. *Neurosurgery,* Vol.50, No.4, (2002 Apr), pp.(850-5), ISSN 0418-396X.

Malik, K. & Benzon, HT. (2008). Radiofrequency applications to dorsal root ganglia: A literature review. *Anesthesiology,* Vol.109, No.3, (2008 Sep), pp.(527-42), ISSN 0003-3022.

Munglani, R. (1999). The longer term effect of pulsed radiofrequency for neuropathic pain. *Pain,* Vol.80, No.1-2, (1999 Mar), pp.(437-9), ISSN 0304-3959.

Niv, D. & Gofeld, M. (2009). Percutaneous neural destructive techniques. In: *Neural Blockade in clinical anesthesia and pain medicine,* 4th edition, Cousins, MJ., Carr, DB., Horlocker, TT., & Bridenbaugh, PO., pp.(991-1035), Lippincott Williams & Wilkins, ISBN 978-0-7817-7388-1, Philadelphia, USA.

Organ, LW. (1976-1977) Electrophysiologic principles of radiofrequency lesion making. *Appl Neurophysiol,* Vol.39, No.2, pp.(69-76), ISSN 0302-2773.

Pockett, S. (1995). Spinal cord synaptic plasticity and chronic pain. *Anesth Analg,* Vol.80, No.1, (1995 Jan), pp.(173-9), ISSN 0003-2999.

Podhajsky, RJ., Sekiguchi, Y., Kikuchi, S. & Myers, RR. (2005). The histologic effects of pulsed and continuous radiofrequency lesions at 42 degrees C to rat dorsal root ganglion and sciatic nerve. *Spine (Phila Pa 1976),* Vol.30, No.9, (2005 May), pp.(1008-13), ISSN 0362-2436.

Protasoni, M., Reguzzoni, M., Sangiorgi, S., Reverberi, C., Borsani, E., Rodella, LF., Dario, A., Tomei, G. & Dell'orbo, C. (2009). Pulsed radiofrequency effects on the lumbar ganglion of the rat dorsal root: A morphological light and transmission electron microscopy study at acute stage. *Eur Spine J,* Vol.18, No.4, (2009 Apr), pp.(473-8), ISSN 0940-6719.

Racz, GB. & Ruiz-Lopez, R. (2006). Radiofrequency procedures. *Pain Pract,* Vol.6, No.1, (2006 Mar), pp.(46-50), ISSN 1530-7085.

Rathmell, JP. (2009). Complications in Pain Medicine. In: *Neural Blockade in clinical anesthesia and pain medicine, 4th edition,* Cousins, MJ., Carr, DB., Horlocker, TT., & Bridenbaugh, PO., pp. (1223-1267), Lippincott Williams & Wilkins, ISBN 978-0-7817-7388-1, Philadelphia, USA.

Romundstad, L. & Stubhaug, A. (2007). Glucocorticoids for acute and persistent postoperative neuropathic pain: What is the evidence? *Anesthesiology,* Vol.107, No.3, (2007 Sep), pp.(371-3), ISSN 0003-3022.

Sandkühler, J., Chen, JG., Cheng, G. & Randić, M. (1997). Low-frequency stimulation of afferent adelta-fibers induces long-term depression at primary afferent synapses with substantia gelatinosa neurons in the rat. *J Neurosci,* Vol.17, No.16, (1997 Aug), pp.(6483-91), ISSN 0270-6474.

Simopoulos, TT., Kraemer, J., Nagda, JV., Aner, M. & Bajwa, ZH. (2008). Response to pulsed and continuous radiofrequency lesioning of the dorsal root ganglion and segmental nerves in patients with chronic lumbar radicular pain. *Pain Physician,* Vol. 11, No. 2 (2008 March/April), pp.(137-44), ISSN 1533-3159.

Slappendel, R., Crul, BJ., Braak, GJ., Geurts, JW., Booij, LH., Voerman, VF. & De Boo, T. (1997). The efficacy of radiofrequency lesioning of the cervical spinal dorsal root ganglion in a double blinded randomized study: No difference between 40°C and 67°C treatments. *Pain,* Vol.73, No.2, (1997 Nov), pp.(159-63), ISSN 0304-3959.

Sluijter, ME., Cosman ER., Rittman, WB. & Van Kleef, M. (1998). The effects of pulsed radiofrequency fields applied to the dorsal root ganglion—A preliminary report. *Pain Clin,* Vol.11, No.2, pp.(109-118).

Sluijter, ME. (2001). *Radiofrequency Part 1,* FlivoPress, ISBN 3-909 441-00-9, Meggen, Switzerland.

Smith, HP., Mcwhorter, JM. & Challa, VR. (1981). Radiofrequency neurolysis in a clinical model. Neuropathological correlation. *J Neurosurg,* Vol.55, No.2, (1981 Aug), pp.(246-53), ISSN 0022-3085.

Stolker, RJ., Vervest, AC. & Groen, GJ. (1994). The treatment of chronic thoracic segmental pain by radiofrequency percutaneous partial rhizotomy. *J Neurosurg,* Vol.80, No.6, (1994 June), pp.(986-92), ISSN 0022-3085.

Taha, JM. & Tew, JM., Jr. (1996). Comparison of surgical treatments for trigeminal neuralgia: Reevaluation of radiofrequency rhizotomy. *Neurosurgery,* Vol.38, No.5, (1996 May), pp.(865-71), ISSN 0148-396X.

Tun, K., Cemil, B., Gurcay, AG., Kaptanoglu, E., Sargon, MF., Tekdemir, I., Comert, A. & Kanpolat, Y. (2009). Ultrastructural evaluation of pulsed radiofrequency and conventional radiofrequency lesions in rat sciatic nerve. *Surg Neurol,* Vol.72, No.5, (2009 Nov), pp.(496-500), ISSN 0090-3019.

Uchida, K. (2009). Radiofrequency treatment of the thoracic paravertebral nerve combined with glucocorticoid for refractory neuropathic pain following breast cancer surgery. *Pain Physician,* Vol. 12, No. 4, (2009 July/Aug), pp (E277-83), ISSN 2150-1149.

Uematsu, S., Udvarhelyi, GB., Benson, DW. & Siebens, AA. (1974). Percutaneous radiofrequency rhizotomy. *Surg Neurol,* Vol.2, No.5, (1974 Sep), pp.(319-25), ISSN 0090-3019.

Van Kleef, M., Barendse, GA., Dingemans, WA., Wingen, C., Lousberg, R., De Lange, S. & Sluijter, ME. (1995). Effects of producing a radiofrequency lesion adjacent to the dorsal root ganglion in patients with thoracic segmental pain. *Clin J Pain,* Vol.11, No.4, (1995 Dec), pp.(325-32), ISSN 0749-8047.

Van Kleef, M., Liem, L., Lousberg, R., Barendse, G., Kessels, F. & Sluijter, M. (1996). Radiofrequency lesion adjacent to the dorsal root ganglion for cervicobrachial pain: A prospective double blind randomized study. *Neurosurgery,* Vol.38, No.6, (1996 Jun), pp.(1127-31), ISSN 0148-396X.

Van Zundert, J., De Louw, AJ., Joosten, EA., Kessels, AG., Honig, W., Dederen, P J., Veening, JG., Vles, JS. & Van Kleef, M. (2005). Pulsed and continuous radiofrequency current adjacent to the cervical dorsal root ganglion of the rat induces late cellular activity in the dorsal horn. *Anesthesiology,* Vol.102, No.1, (2005 Jan), pp.(125-31), ISSN 0003-3022.

Van Zundert, J., Patijn, J., Kessels, A., Lame, I., Van Suijlekom, H. & Van Kleef, M. (2007). Pulsed radiofrequency adjacent to the cervical dorsal root ganglion in chronic cervical radicular pain: A double blind sham controlled randomized clinical trial. *Pain,* Vol.127, No.1-2, (2007 Jan), pp.(173-82), ISSN 0304-3959.